Springer
Tokyo
Berlin
Heidelberg
New York
Barcelona
Hong Kong
London
Milan
Paris

H.E. Takahashi, T. Morita
T. Hotta, A. Ogose (Eds.)

Operative Treatment of Pelvic Tumors

With 183 Figures

Springer

Hideaki E. Takahashi, M.D., Ph.D.
President
Niigata University of Health and Welfare
1398 Shimami-cho, Niigata 950-3198, Japan

Tetsuro Morita, M.D., Ph.D.
Chief
Department of Orthopedic Surgery
Niigata Cancer Center Hospital
2-15-3 Kawagishi-cho, Niigata 951-8566, Japan

Tetsuo Hotta, M.D., Ph.D.
Associate Professor
Operating Room Division
Niigata University Medical Hospital
1-754 Asahimachi-dori, Niigata 951-8510, Japan

Akira Ogose, M.D., Ph.D.
Senior Assistant Professor
Division of Orthopedic Surgery, Department of Regenerative and Transplant Medicine,
Course for Biological Functions and Medical Control,
Graduate School of Medical and Dental Science, Niigata University
1-757 Asahimachi-dori, Niigata 951-8510, Japan

Cover: T2-weighted MR imaging. The tumor showed a very high intensity image and arose from the body of S3 (*arrows*)

Library of Congress Cataloging-in-Publication Data
Operative treatment of pelvic tumors / H.E. Takahashi ... [et al.] (eds.).
p. ; cm.
Includes bibliographical references and index.

ISBN 978-4-431-66867-1 ISBN 978-4-431-66865-7 (eBook)
DOI 10.1007/978-4-431-66865-7

1. Pelvis—Cancer—Surgery. 2. Pelvis—Cancer—Treatment. I. Takahashi, Hideaki, 1933–
[DNLM: 1. Pelvic Neoplasms—surgery. 2. Pelvis—surgery. 3. Surgical Procedures, Operative. WE 750 O61 2002]
RD669.5 .O745 2002
616.99′496059—dc21

2002029171

Printed on acid-free paper

Softcover reprint of the hardcover 1st edition 2003

Typesetting: SNP Best-set Typesetter Ltd., Hong Kong

SPIN: 10855986

This book is dedicated
to Professor Crawford Jennings Campbell,
a superb orthopedic surgeon and inspirational teacher,
in remembrance of his many acts of generosity.
This book would not have been published
without Professor Campbell's introduction for the authors to,
and his enthusiasm for, bone tumor pathology.

Preface

This book presents our experience in the operative treatment of bone and soft-tissue tumors arising in and around the pelvis, from 1970 to 1999 in the Department of Orthopedic Surgery at the Niigata University Medical Hospital.

Histological diagnoses included both benign and malignant tumors. Surgical planning was difficult to perform in our early experience in operative treatment, when only angiography and barium enemas were in use. In the meantime, computed tomography scanning and magnetic resonance imaging became available. Subsequent improvement in the quality of these images made three-dimensional surgical planning for pelvic tumor removal much easier. Such progress in diagnostic methodologies, together with advancements in microsurgical techniques, methods of irradiation, and various adjuvant chemotherapies has led to significant improvements in the treatment of pelvic tumors. Furthermore, these advancements were enhanced by the availability of various conventional and custom-made endoprostheses, plates and screws, spinal instruments, and external fixators made of 316L stainless steel, titanium, high-density polyethylene, and ceramics.

Because sacral tumors are so silent and symptomless, they may grow to a large size and be difficult to excise. Removal of sacral tumors might make subjective symptoms worse because the sacrum contains the cauda equina. Excision of a tumor that involves the ilium and sacroiliac joint may interrupt the structural stability of the pelvic ring. A tumor affecting the hip joint may require reconstruction to re-establish the function of the hip and to provide stability for gait after operative treatment. Each case of treatment of a pelvic tumor has to be considered individually. The quality of life of the patient after possible surgery must be taken into account.

The senior editor and author (H.E.T.) of this book, when he was an orthopedic fellow from 1959 to 1960, had the opportunity to learn about bone pathology from the late Dr. Crawford J. Campbell at the Albany Medical Center Hospital, Albany, New York. Two other authors and/or editors of this book were also trained in Albany (H.S.) and Boston (T.M.) by him. Dr. Campbell was a corresponding member of the Japanese Orthopaedic Association. At that time, large sections of bone tumors were made at Dr. Mary Sherman's bone pathology laboratory in Chicago, and were arranged and classified by Dr. Campbell and the senior author at the office on New Scotland Avenue in Albany. Thus, the senior author became interested in bone pathology. In 1982, Professor Campbell visited Niigata and made rounds in our ward, observing our pelvic tumor cases. He suggested that we publish a series of case reports, because each case exhibited a particular point of interest in the treatment of pelvic tumors.

This challenge was finally realized with the completion of this book. Seventeen illustrative cases in chapter 10 and a case with a free vascularized foot–ankle joint graft in chapter 6 are included to present the outcome of the operative treatment of pelvic tumors. We hope that our experience will be useful for the readers of this book, especially senior orthopedic residents and young oncology surgeons, who will be responsible for the future surgical treatment of pelvic tumors.

The authors are most grateful to Professor Emeritus Tatsuya Tajima, who has always encouraged us in treating bone tumors. We are also very grateful to the senior orthopedic residents who took direct care of our patients. Without their efforts, these patients could not have been treated. We would like to express our sincere gratitude to the Alumni Society of the Orthopedic Department of Niigata University for their strong support that made this publication possible. We owe a deep debt of gratitude to Ms. Tomoko Yuasa, who provided superb secretarial support, and to Mr. William Lew, for his expert editing. Finally, we would like to thank the staff of Springer-Verlag Tokyo for their patience and continuous efforts in compiling the manuscripts for the publication of this book.

Hideaki E. Takahashi
Senior Editor and Author
November 2001

Contents

Chapter 5: Approach

Chapter 6: Reconstruction

Chapter 7: Related Topics

Chapter 8: Complications

Chapter 9: Outcomes

Chapter 10: Case Presentations

Contributors

Takeshi Higuchi, M.D.
Chief, Department of Radiology, Niigata City General Hospital, 2-6-1 Shichikuyama, Niigata 950-8739, Japan
*Department of Radiology, Niigata University School of Medicine, 1-757 Asahimachi-dori, Niigata 951-8510, Japan

Tetsuo Hotta, M.D., Ph.D.
Associate Professor, Operating Room Division, Niigata University Medical Hospital, 1-754 Asahimachi-dori, Niigata 951-8510, Japan
*Department of Orthopedic Surgery, Niigata University School of Medicine, 1-757 Asahimachi-dori, Niigata 951-8510, Japan

Yoshiya Z. Inoue, M.D., Ph.D.
Vice-Chairman, Department of Orthopedic Surgery, Seirei Hamamatsu General Hospital, 2-12-12 Sumiyoshi, Hamamatsu, Shizuoka 430-8558, Japan

Tetsuro Morita, M.D., Ph.D.
Chief, Department of Orthopedic Surgery, Niigata Cancer Center Hospital, 2-15-3 Kawagishi-cho, Niigata 951-8566, Japan

Akira Ogose, M.D., Ph.D.
Senior Assistant Professor, Division of Orthopedic Surgery, Department of Regenerative and Transplant Medicine, Course for Biological Functions and Medical Control, Graduate School of Medical and Dental Science, Niigata University, 1-757 Asahimachi-dori, Niigata 951-8510, Japan
*Department of Orthopedic Surgery, Niigata University School of Medicine, 1-757 Asahimachi-dori, Niigata 951-8510, Japan

Hidehiko Saito, M.D., Ph.D.
Hospital Vice-Director, Chief, Department of Orthopedic Surgery, Seirei Hamamatsu General Hospital, 2-12-12 Sumiyoshi, Hamamatsu, Shizuoka 430-8558, Japan

Minoru Shibata, M.D., Ph.D.
Professor, Division of Plastic and Reconstructive Surgery, Niigata University Medical Hospital, 1-754 Asahimachi-dori, Niigata 951-8510, Japan

Hideaki E. Takahashi, M.D., Ph.D.
President, Niigata University of Health and Welfare, 1398 Shimami-cho, Niigata 950-3198, Japan
*Professor and Chair, Department of Orthopedic Surgery, Niigata University School of Medicine, 1-757 Asahimachi-dori, Niigata 951-8510, Japan

Takeshi Tojo, M.D., Ph.D.
Chief, Department of Orthopaedic Surgery, Niigata Prefectural Central Hospital, 205 Shin-nan-cho, Johetsu, Niigata 943-0192, Japan

*Former affiliation and address (as of March 1999)

Introduction

Tetsuro Morita

Surgical treatment of pelvic tumors, especially malignant tumors, is difficult for several reasons. First, in many cases there are no symptoms until the tumor has grown to a large size. Surgeons frequently encounter a massive chondrosarcoma, giant cell tumor, or chordoma of the pelvis. In such cases of tumors with extended growth, a wide margin can seldom be obtained because of the anatomy of the pelvis. Second, orthopedic surgeons, in general, are not familiar with the anatomy of the vessels and nerves in the pelvic cavity. In addition, pelvic tumors are relatively rare, and orthopedic surgeons do not have many opportunities to become skilled in pelvic tumor surgery. Massive bleeding of over 5000 ml is often encountered, and the operative time is usually very long. Third, a histological diagnosis is difficult because often a biopsy specimen cannot easily be obtained. Open biopsy often leads to contamination of the tumor tissue, massive bleeding, or unnecessary free flaps.

This textbook has been written to assist in the training of senior residents and young specialists in musculoskeletal tumor surgery. It is a manual that presents the practical aspects of pelvic tumor surgery. The contents are based on actual experiences, including some trial procedures which failed. The importance of the imaging examination, the timing and an appropriate procedure for obtaining a biopsy (including aspiration cytology), the practical aspects of preparation for surgery, the program of postoperative care, and the surgical techniques available are described in detail, with abundant illustrations and photographs. Typical procedures and topics of interest are explained in the chapter containing case reports.

Surgical planning is the most important factor in pelvic tumor surgery. All imaging examinations should be carried out before any surgical intervention, including biopsy. Then a histological diagnosis can be made by aspiration cytology or open biopsy. We recommend aspiration cytology. Obtaining a biopsy is particularly difficult with pelvic tumors. The choice of timing and the appropriate procedure are described in the chapter on biopsy. After the tumor has been diagnosed, the surgical margin should be determined according to the grade of the tumor. At this time, adjuvant therapy should also be considered for high-grade tumors such as an osteosarcoma or Ewing's sarcoma. Current thinking is that neoadjuvant and adjuvant chemotherapy is essential for these tumors. Preoperative radiation therapy may be used for Ewing's sarcoma. However, the efficacy of this therapy is still controversial. Postoperative radiation therapy or brachytherapy may be effective in cases with an inadequate surgical margin. The preparations before surgery are also important. Can the rectum be preserved? Is urinary diversion necessary? Is vascular reconstruction needed? How much bleeding is expected? These questions must be settled before surgery. Consultations should be carried out with a general surgeon, a urologist, and a vascular surgeon, when necessary. The procedures for surgical preparation are described in the chapter on preparation. It is helpful to simulate the surgery using paper templates in order to visualize and understand the three-dimensional anatomy. The surgical approaches for pelvic tumors are complicated. These approaches are described according to the type of tumor in the context of actual cases, complete with illustrations and photographs. Planning for the reconstruction of the site of tumor removal is also very important, especially in the hip and sacroiliac joints. Actual methods of reconstruction are described in the chapter on reconstruction and in the case reports.

An orthopedic surgeon who performs surgery on pelvic tumors must be skilled in basic surgical techniques and be intimately aware of the anatomy of the pelvis. Take your courage in both hands, and you will accomplish the difficult task of pelvic surgery. We hope this textbook will be helpful to young surgeons who become involved in pelvic tumor surgery.

Chapter 1
Surgical Anatomy

Normal Anatomy and Magnetic Resonance Appearance of the Pelvis

TAKESHI HIGUCHI

Summary. The normal pelvic anatomy and its radiological appearance on magnetic resonance imaging (MRI) are described, including the blood vessels, nerves, pelvic organs, sacrum, pelvic floor, and ligaments of the sacroiliac joint, with many images. MRI is a very useful evaluation tool both before and after pelvic surgery.

Key words. Pelvic anatomy, Magnetic resonance imaging (MRI)

Blood Vessels

Arteries of the Pelvis

The abdominal aorta divides into the right and left common iliac arteries at the level of the fourth lumbar vertebra. Each common iliac artery runs anterior to the common iliac vein, and divides into the external iliac artery and internal iliac artery at the level of the lower end of the fifth lumbar vertebra. The median sacral artery arises from the aorta at its bifurcation, and runs straight down the midline.

Each external iliac artery (Figs. 1f,k, 2, 3) descends along the psoas major muscle to the level of the inguinal ligament. The inferior epigastric artery and deep iliac circumflex artery originate from the external iliac artery just above or just below the inguinal ligament.

The branches of the internal iliac artery supply most of the pelvic organs except the ovaries, rectum, and posterior pelvic wall. The internal iliac artery (Figs. 1f, 2, 3) passes down into the pelvis at the upper margin of the greater sciatic foramen.

In spin-echo magnetic resonance (MR) images, blood vessels with a normal flow velocity typically appear as areas void of any signal. However, the signal intensity from blood depends upon flow direction and velocity in addition to the MR imaging parameters (Hricak and Carrington 1991).

The branches of the internal iliac artery are clinically divided into the visceral branches and the parietal branches.

Visceral Branches of the Internal Iliac Artery

The superior vesical arteries, which arise from the terminal portion of the umbilical artery, supply the superior part of the urinary bladder. The uterine artery in the

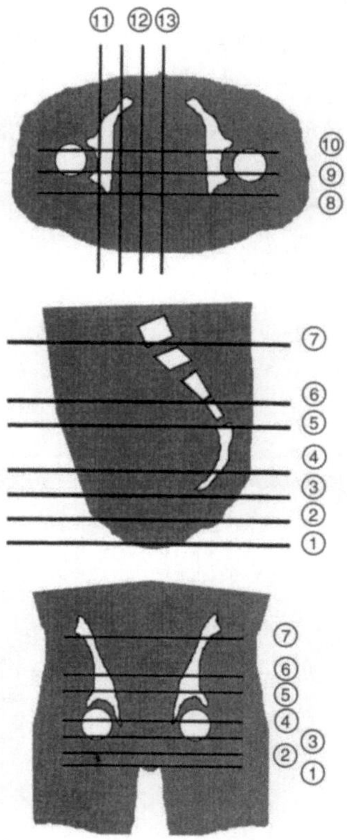

a

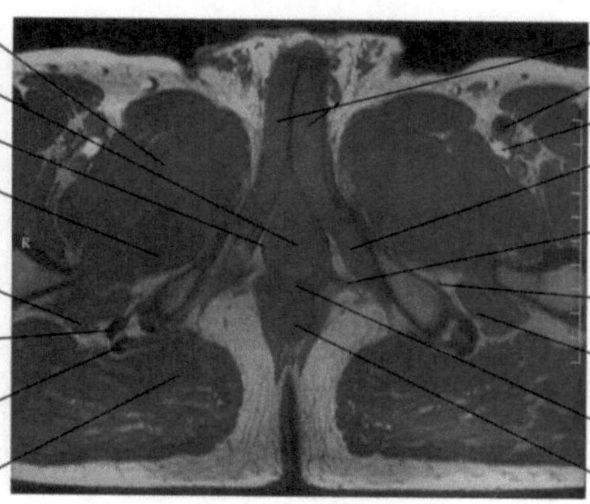

b

FIG. 1. Magnetic resonance images showing the anatomy of the pelvis. **a** The numbers indicate the planes along which the images in each part of the figure were taken: 1, **b**; 2, **c**,**i**; 3, **d**,**j**; 4, **e**,**k**; 5, **f**; 6, **g**; 7, **h**; 8, **l**; 9, **m**; 10, **n**; 11, **o**; 12, **p**; 13, **q**,**r**. **b–h** Axial T1-weighted images (repetiton time (TR) = 550 ms, echo time (TE) = 12 ms) of the pelvis of a 30-year-old male. **i–k** Axial T2-weighted images (TR = 3500 ms, TE = 96 ms) of the pelvis of a 28-year-old female. **l–n** Coronal T1-weighted images (TR = 550 ms, TE = 12 ms) of the pelvis of a 30-year-old male. **o–q** Sagittal T1-weighted images (TR = 550 ms, TE = 12 ms) of the pelvis of a 30-year-old male. **r** Sagittal image (TR = 3500 ms, TE = 96 ms) of the pelvis of a 28-year-old female

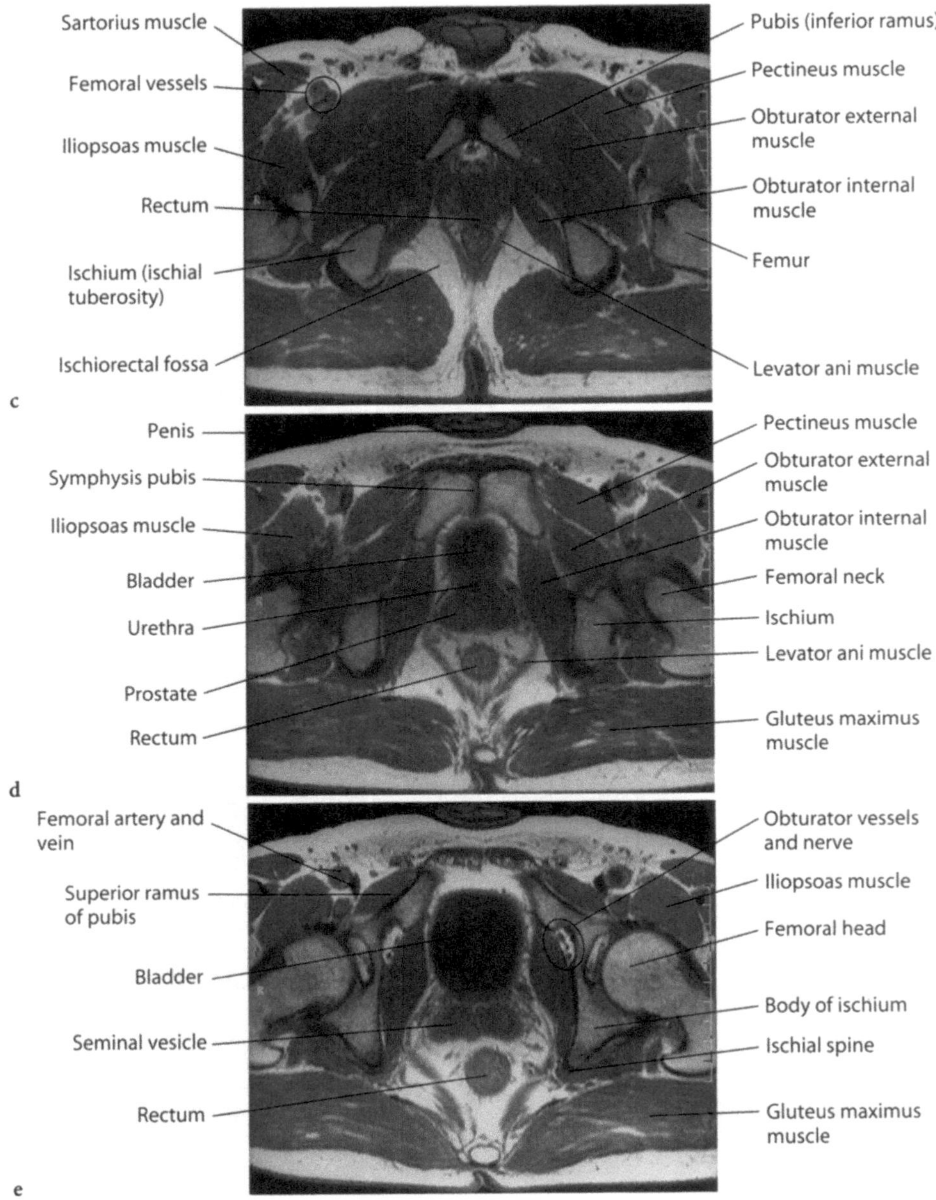

FIG. 1. *Continued*

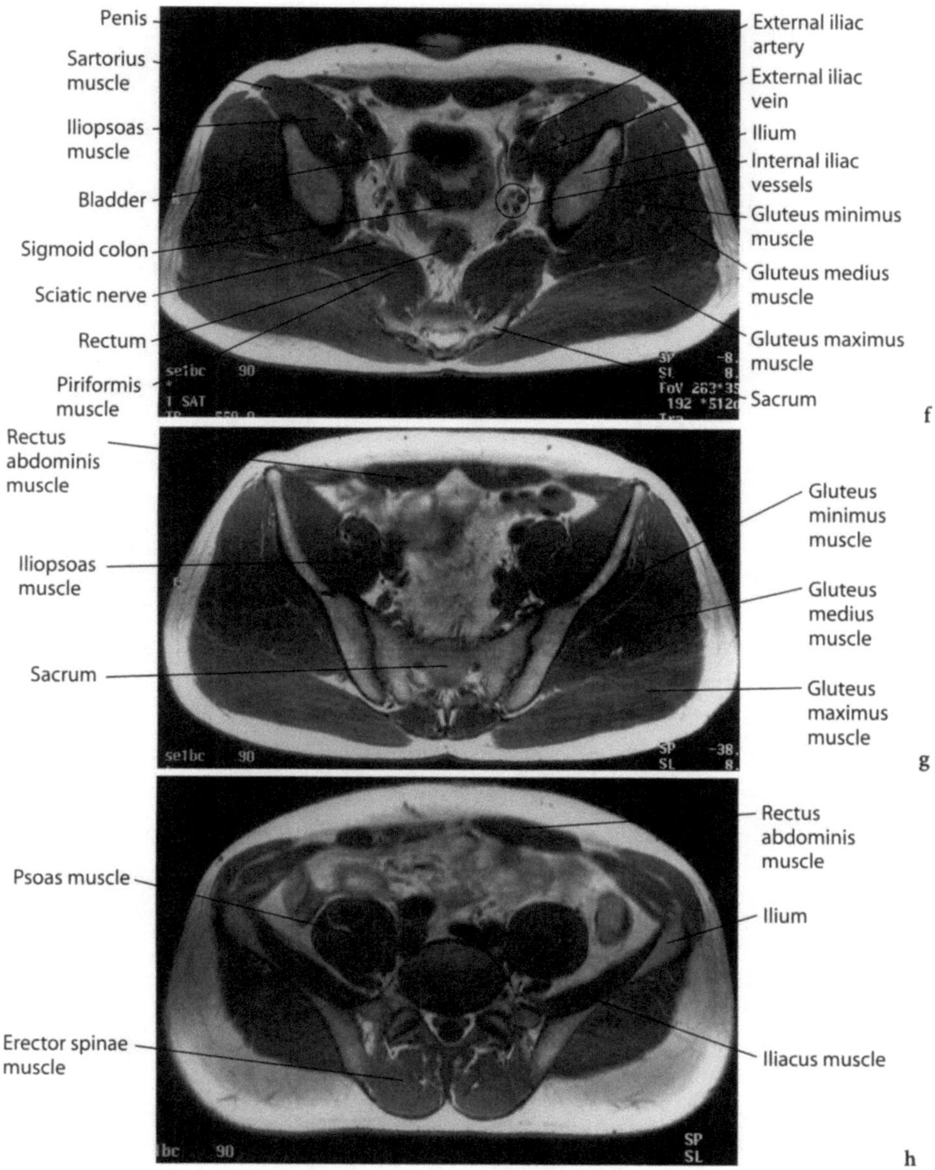

FIG. 1. *Continued*

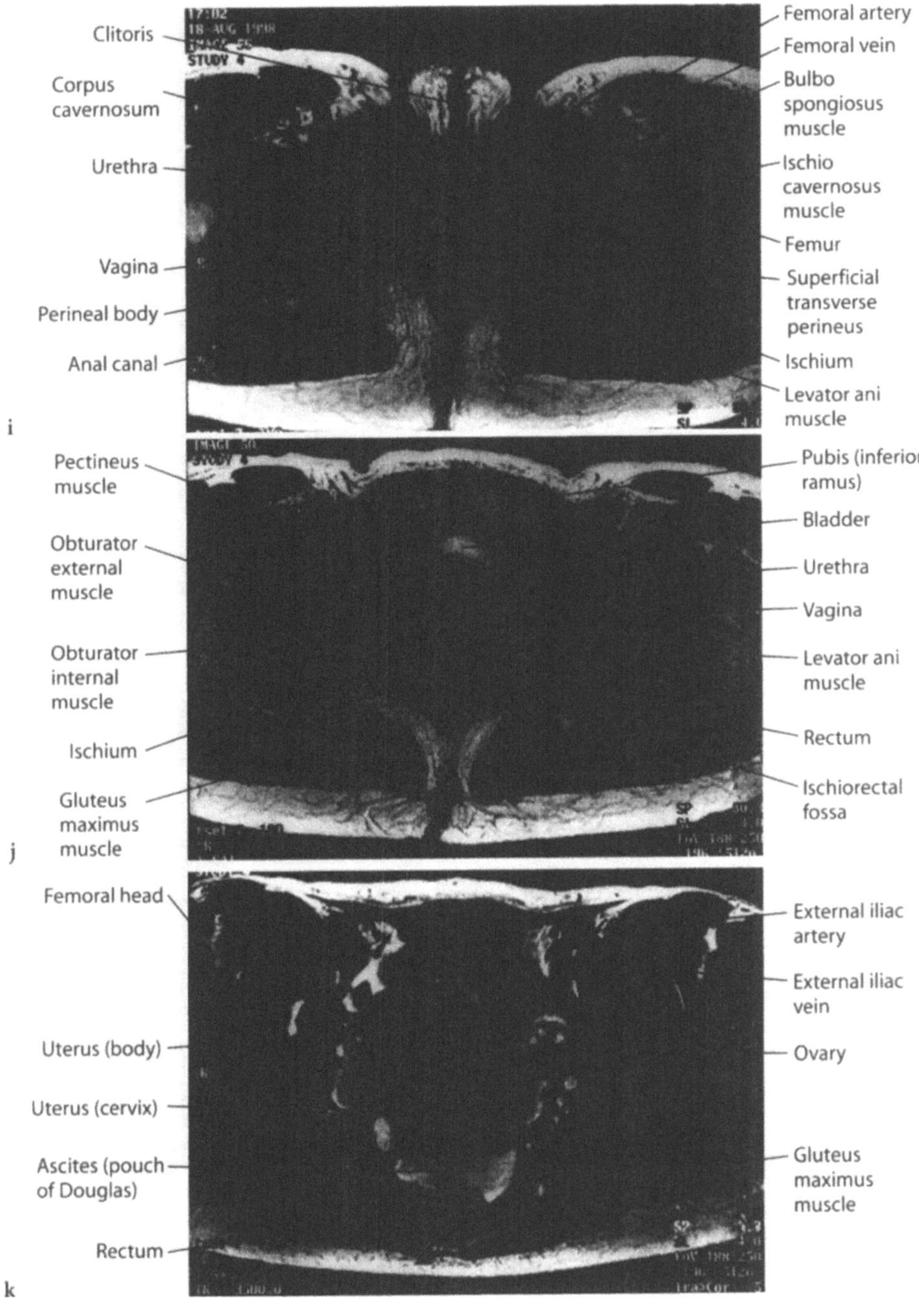

FIG. 1. *Continued*

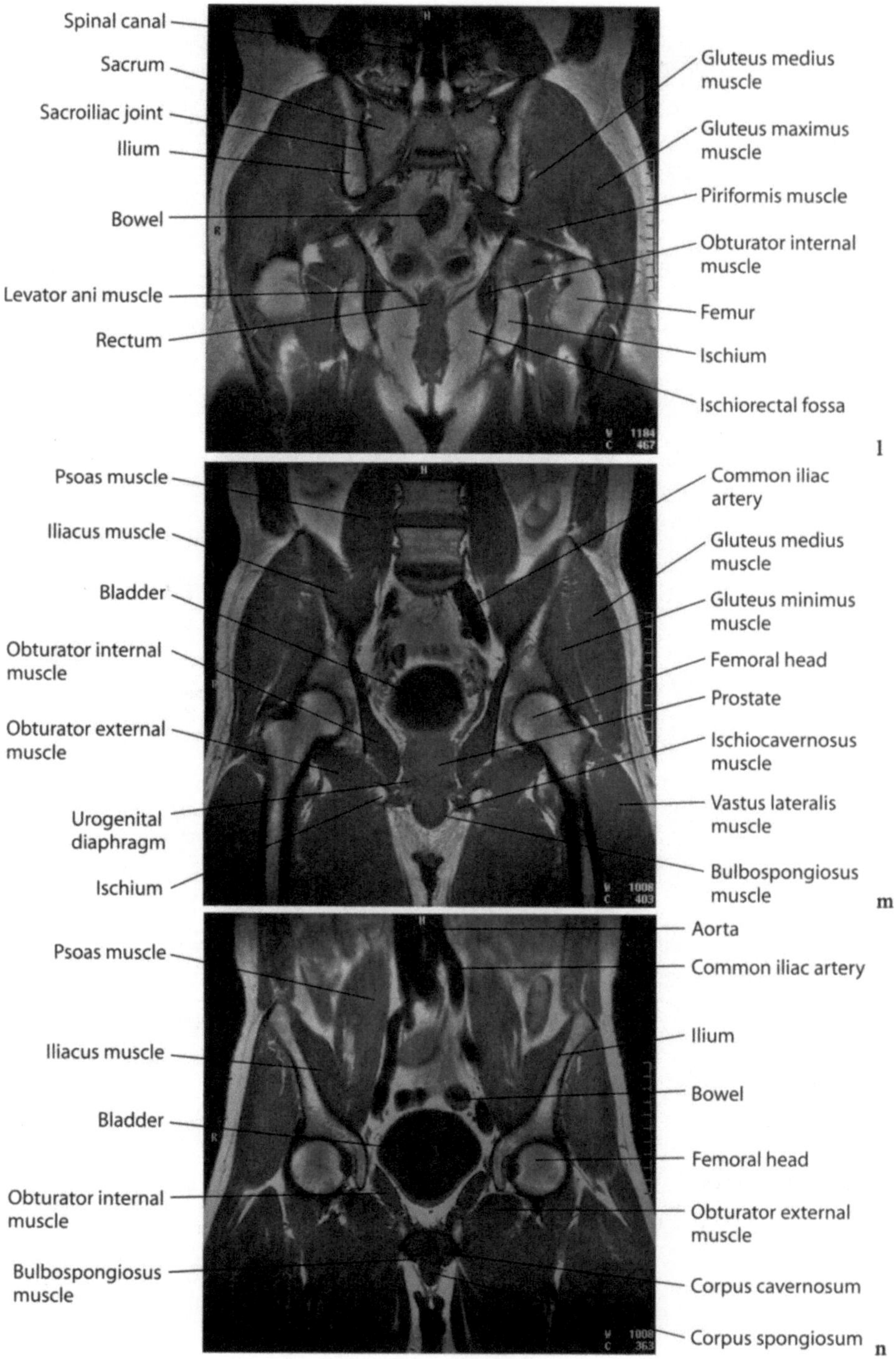

FIG. 1. *Continued*

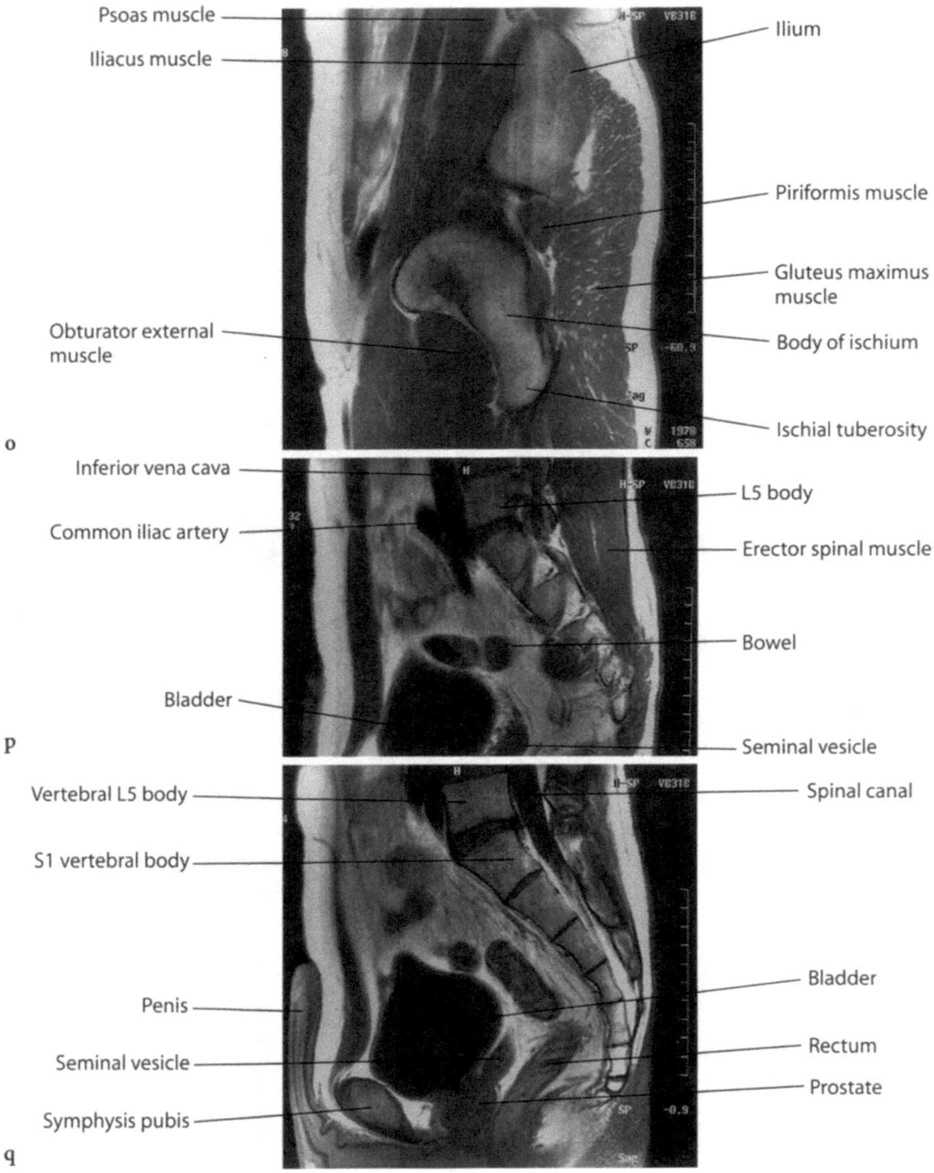

FIG. 1. *Continued*

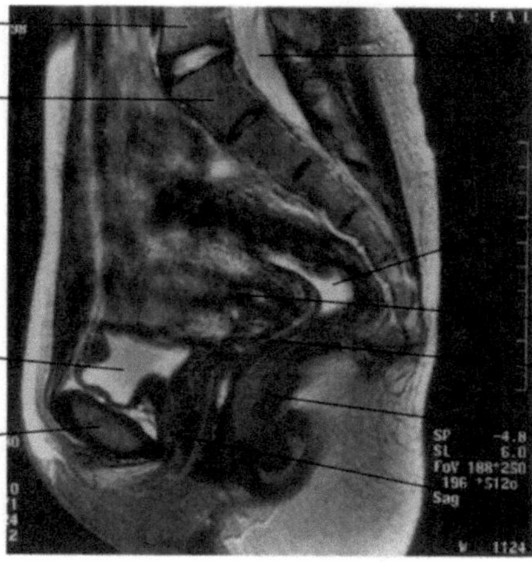

r

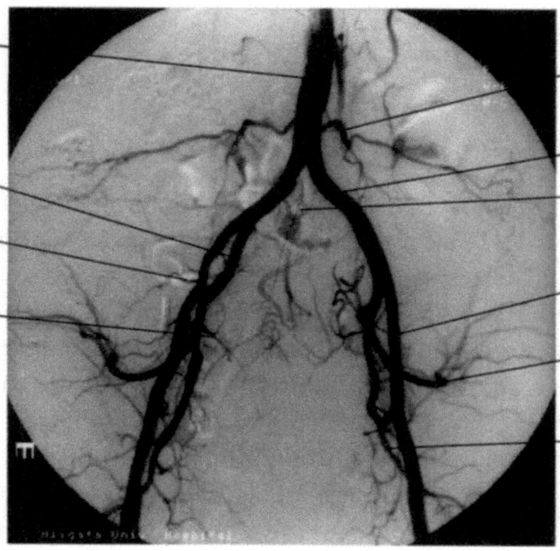

FIG. 2. Arteriogram of the iliac arteries and their branches in a female, using digital subtraction angiography (anterior view)

female runs on the pelvic floor and supplies the cervix and corpus of the uterus, and the ovaries. The branches for the ovary anastomose with the ovarian artery. The vaginal artery in the female arises not only from the uterine artery, but also directly from the internal iliac arteries. The inferior vesical artery extends to the lower portion of the bladder, the prostate in the male, and the vagina in the female. The middle rectal artery arises from the inferior vesical artery or internal pudendal artery, and reaches the rectum, where it anastomoses with the inferior rectal arteries.

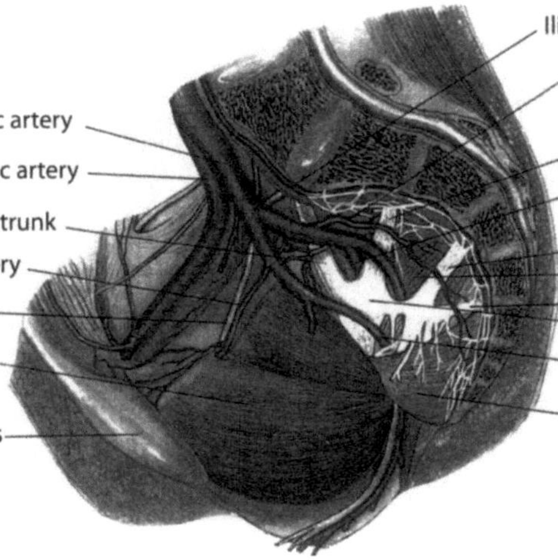

FIG. 3. Branches of the internal iliac artery and sacral plexus (midsagittal view of the right pelvic wall). The sacral plexus lies on the posterolateral pelvic wall in front of the piriformis muscle

Parietal Branches of the Internal Iliac Artery

The iliolumbar artery (Figs. 2, 3) ascends laterally, anterior to the sacroiliac joint. It divides into the lumbar and iliac branches behind the psoas major muscle. The lateral sacral artery (Figs. 2, 3) descends in front of the sacrum, medial to the anterior sacral foramina, and anastomoses with the medial sacral artery. The superior gluteal artery (Figs. 2, 3) is the largest branch of the internal iliac artery. It exits the pelvis by the greater sciatic foramen, above the piriformis muscle, and reaches each gluteal muscle. The obturator artery (Figs. 1e, 3) extends anteriorly on the lateral pelvic wall to the obturator foramen. It exits the pelvis through the obturator canal, together with the obturator nerve. The inferior gluteal artery (Fig. 2) supplies the buttock and thigh. It descends anterior to the sacral plexus and piriformis muscle, and exits the pelvis by the greater sciatic foramen. The internal pudendal artery (Fig. 3) is the main feeder of the perineum. It exits the pelvis through the greater sciatic foramen, and enters the gluteal region. It then curves around the dorsum of the ischial spine and enters the pelvis again through the lesser sciatic foramen.

Veins of the Pelvis

The external iliac vein (Fig. 1f,k) is the proximal communication of the femoral vein. It ascends to the pelvic brim, and terminates anterior to the sacroiliac joint by joining the internal iliac vein to form the common iliac vein. Blood from the gluteal region, perineum, pelvic wall, and pelvic organs concentrates in the internal iliac vein (Fig. 1f). The internal iliac vein ascends along the medial surface of the lateral pelvic wall, posterior to the internal iliac artery.

Nerves

The nerves in the pelvis include the obturator nerve (derived from the lumbar plexus), the sacral plexus (including its parasympathetic branches), the terminal portion of the sympathetic trunk, and the pelvic autonomic plexuses (Hall-Craggs 1985). All pelvic organs receive autonomic nerves which originate from the right and left pelvic (inferior hypogastric) plexuses.

The obturator nerve (Figs. 1e, 3) originates from the lumbar plexus (L2–4). It emerges from the medial border of the psoas muscle, runs in front of the sacroiliac joint into the pelvis, and then descends along the lateral pelvic wall to the obturator foramen. It passes through the foramen along with the obturator vessels, and supplies the muscles of the medial thigh.

The sacral plexus (Fig. 3) supplies the lower limbs, pelvic wall, pelvic floor, and perineum. It lies on the posterolateral pelvic wall in front of the piriformis muscle, and is covered by the parietal pelvic fascia. This plexus is formed by the lumbosacral trunk (part of the fourth and all of the fifth lumbar ventral rami) (Fig. 3), the first to third sacral ventral rami, and part of the fourth sacral ventral rami. The major branches of this nerve exit the pelvis through the greater sciatic foramen.

In T1-weighted MR images, the fourth lumbar to fourth sacral nerves and the sacral plexus have a signal intensity similar to that of muscle. The signal intensity of these nerves and plexus in T2-weighted images is slightly higher compared with that of muscle (Gierada et al. 1993). The sacral coronal plane, which is parallel to the long axis of the sacrum, is best for a visualization of the bony sacrum, sacral foramina, and proximal first sacral to fourth sacral nerve roots (Blake et al. 1996).

Autonomic Nervous System

The autonomic system in the pelvis plays an essential role in the control of defecation, micturition, and sexual intercourse (Hall-Craggs 1985). It is important that the surgeon understand the anatomy of the pelvic autonomic system in order to avoid impairment of sexual or bladder function.

The main route of the sympathetic fibers which enter the pelvis is the superior hypogastric plexus. The branches from this plexus continue to the right and left hypogastric nerves. The hypogastric nerves then continue to each pelvic plexus. The pelvic splanchnic nerves, which originate from the branches of the anterior rami of the second to fourth sacral nerves, constitute the sacral portion of the parasympathetic system.

The right and left pelvic plexuses receive contributions from the superior hypogastric plexus, sacral splanchnic nerves of the sacral sympathetic trunk, and parasympathetic fibers from the pelvic splanchnic nerves (Hall-Craggs 1985). The pelvic plexuses are situated in the extraperitoneal connective tissue between the peritoneum and the levator ani muscle. Each plexus is located lateral to the rectum, at the level of the lower third of the rectum, and just above the levator ani muscles (Pearl et al. 1986). The anterior ends of the plexuses innervate the posterior portion of the urinary bladder. The visceral branches of the internal iliac artery cross the pelvic plexus, since the plexus is medial to the artery. This is one of the reasons for the difficulties encountered in surgery on the pelvic organs.

Nerves of the Gluteal Region

The superior gluteal nerve (L4–5, S1) originates from the sacral plexus and exits the pelvis at the greater sciatic foramen, above the piriformis muscle. The superior gluteal nerve runs laterally between the gluteus medius and gluteus minimus, and supplies these muscles. Finally, it extends to the tensor fasciae latae muscles. The inferior gluteal nerve (L5, S1–2) is located below the piriformis muscle and innervates the gluteus maximus muscle. The pudendal nerve (S2–4) enters the gluteal region through the greater sciatic foramen, below the piriformis muscle, along with the internal pudendal artery. It crosses the ischial spine, and exits the region of the perineum through the lesser sciatic notch. The pudendal nerve supplies the perineum. The sciatic nerve (L4–5, S1–3) (Fig. 1f) is the largest nerve of the lower limbs and the most important structure in the gluteal region. Its branches supply the flexor muscles in the thigh, and all of the muscles in the leg and foot. It passes through the greater sciatic foramen below the piriformis muscle. It is covered by the gluteus maximus muscle in the buttock. As it curves laterally and distally, it is situated midway between the posterior superior iliac spine and ischial tuberosity proximally, and midway between the tip of the greater trochanter and ischial tuberosity distally (Fig. 1c) (Hall-Craggs 1985).

The piriformis muscle is a recognizable landmark that is extremely helpful in locating the sacral plexus and sciatic nerve on computerized axial tomography (CAT) (Lanzieri and Hilal 1984) and MR images.

Pelvic Organs

The sigmoid colon (Fig. 1f) has a sigmoid mesocolon which is attached to the left posterior wall of the pelvic cavity. The blood supply for the sigmoid colon is from the sigmoid artery, which is derived from the inferior mesenteric artery.

The rectum (Fig. 1c–f,j–l,q,r) is located in the posterior part of the pelvic cavity. It begins in front of the third sacral vertebra as a continuation of the sigmoid colon. The rectum descends, with an anteroposterior curve, along the anterior surface of the sacrum. It is continuous with the anal canal at the level of the pelvic floor. The main blood supply for the rectum is from the superior rectal artery, which is derived from the inferior mesenteric artery. The lower part of the rectum is supplied by the inferior rectal artery. In T1-weighted MR images, the rectum has a low-to-medium signal intensity, and is well delineated by the surrounding high signal intensity of the perirectal fat (Heiken and Lee 1988).

Pelvic Viscera in the Male

The right and left ureters descend along the lateral pelvic wall within the extraperitoneal space in front of the internal iliac arteries. They then turn anteromedially, and run along the superior surface of the levator ani muscle to reach the base of the urinary bladder.

The urinary bladder (Fig. 1d–f,m,n,p,q) is situated posterior and superior to the pubis, between the peritoneum and the pelvic floor. Its lateral surfaces are in contact with the fasciae of the internal obturator muscles above and the levator ani muscles below. In the male, the superior surface of the bladder is covered by the peritoneum, and the posterior surface of the bladder is in contact with the seminal vesicles and the terminal portion of the ductus deferens. In T2-weighted MR images, the urinary bladder wall appears as a low-intensity line surrounded medially by high-intensity urine, and laterally and superiorly by high-intensity fat (Heiken and Lee 1988).

The ductus deferens (vas deferens) begins at the epididymal tail and enters the lesser pelvis through the inguinal canal. It runs along the lateral pelvic wall in the extraperitoneal space. It then crosses the obturator nerve and vessels, and the ureter. It finally descends to the base of the prostate to form the ejaculatory duct.

The seminal vesicles (Fig. 1e,p,q) are located within the extraperitoneal fat, posterior to the urinary bladder and superior to the prostate gland. Their posterior surfaces are related to the anterior rectal wall. The signal intensity of normal adult seminal vesicles in T1-weighted spin-echo MR images is similar to, or slightly higher than, that of skeletal muscle, and always higher than urine. In T2-weighted images, the vesicles exhibit signal intensities that can be lower than, similar to, or higher than the signal intensities of urine or fat (Secaf et al. 1991).

The base or superior surface of the prostate (Fig. 1d,m,q) is in contact with the neck of the urinary bladder. The apex of the prostate is located above the urogenital diaphragm. The anterior surface of the prostate is situated near the symphysis pubis, while its posterior surface is closely related to the anterior surface of the rectal ampulla. In T2-weighted MR images, the peripheral and central zones of the prostate can be distinguished. The peripheral zone has a higher signal intensity than the central zone in T2-weighted images (Secaf et al. 1991; Sommer et al. 1986).

The male urethra is divided into prostatic, membranous, and spongy portions. The prostatic urethra descends from the internal urethral orifice to the apex of the prostate, and then passes through the prostate. The membranous urethra runs through the urogenital diaphragm to the bulb of the penis. The membranous urethra is continuous with the spongy urethra, which is the longest portion of the urethra.

Pelvic Viscera in the Female

In females, the upper pelvic portion of the ureters descends along the lateral pelvic wall within the extraperitoneal space, in the same way as in males. The ureters then pass behind the ovary, and are crossed by the uterine artery in the broad ligament of the uterus. On the pelvic floor, they then run anteromedially to enter the urinary bladder.

In the female, the posterior portion of the superior surface of the urinary bladder (Fig. 1j,r) is related to the uterine corpus, and the posterior surface is related to the uterine cervix and anterior wall of the vagina.

The female urethra (Fig. 1r) descends anteriorly from the neck of the urinary bladder to the external ureteral orifice. It runs behind the symphysis pubis, and through the pelvic floor and perineal membrane. In nonenhanced, T1-weighted MR images, the female urethra exhibits a homogeneous medium-intensity signal (similar to that of striated muscle). In T2-weighted images, the zonal anatomy of the urethra can be appreciated (Hricak et al. 1991).

The ovaries (Fig. 1k) are situated on each side of the uterus, close to the lateral pelvic walls. They are attached to the posterosuperior surface of the broad ligaments of the uterus by the mesovarium. They receive their blood supply from the ovarian arteries, which are directly derived from the abdominal aorta. MR imaging has shown normal ovaries in 87% of women of reproductive age (Dooms et al. 1986). The normal ovaries exhibit low-to-medium signal intensity in T1-weighted images, and hyperintensity in T2-weighted images (Dooms et al. 1986). In the T2-weighted images, tiny follicles and stroma are distinguishable within the ovaries (Dooms et al. 1986).

The two uterine tubes lie on each side of the uterus in the upper border of the broad ligament.

The uterus (Fig. 1k,r) is a pear-shaped organ with thick muscular walls. The uterus is divided into the corpus and the cervix. The cervix is the lower third of the uterus, and is narrower and more cylindrical than the corpus. The uterus is situated between the urinary bladder and the rectum, and is normally inclined anteriorly. Thus, the uterine corpus is affected by the volume of the urinary bladder. The uterine corpus protrudes into the pelvic cavity and, except laterally, is covered with peritoneum (Togashi 1993). The cervix is covered with peritoneum only on its posterior aspect (Togashi 1993). The corpus and cervix can be recognized in T2-weighted MR images. Within the corpus, the image of the peripheral myometrium exhibits medium signal intensity, and the endometrium has a very high signal intensity. The myometrium and endometrium are separated by a "junctional zone" or low-intensity line (Heiken and Lee 1988; Hricak 1986). The normal cervix has two separate zones. The cervical epithelium and mucus of the central zone of the cervix exhibits a high-intensity signal. This zone is surrounded by a cylinder of low-intensity fibrous cervical stroma (Heiken and Lee 1988; Hricak 1986).

The vagina (Fig. 1i,j,r) is a muscular tube. The bladder and urethra are located anterior to the vagina, and the rectum and anal canal are situated posteriorly. The upper portion of the vagina lies above the pelvic floor, and the lower portion lies within the perineum. The vagina can be differentiated from surrounding structures in T2-weighted MR images. Its image has a high-intensity center, representing the vaginal epithelium and mucus, and a lower-intensity wall (Hricak 1986).

Sacrum (Pelvic Surface)

The pelvic surface of the sacrum (Fig. 4) is concave in the vertical and horizontal axes, and gives rise to the origins of the piriformis and coccygeus muscles. The sacrum has four paired foramina. The anterior sacral foramina communicate with the sacral canal, and the ventral rami of the upper four sacral spinal nerves exit through the foramina. The anterior surfaces of the first and second sacral bodies, and a portion of the third sacral body, are covered by parietal peritoneum. The rectum is in contact with the remainder of the sacral vertebrae (Williams et al. 1995).

Pelvic Floor

The pelvic cavity is located superior to the pelvic floor, and the perineum is situated inferior to it. The major structure of the pelvic floor is the pelvic diaphragm. The pelvic diaphragm is composed of the levator ani and the coccygeus muscles and their

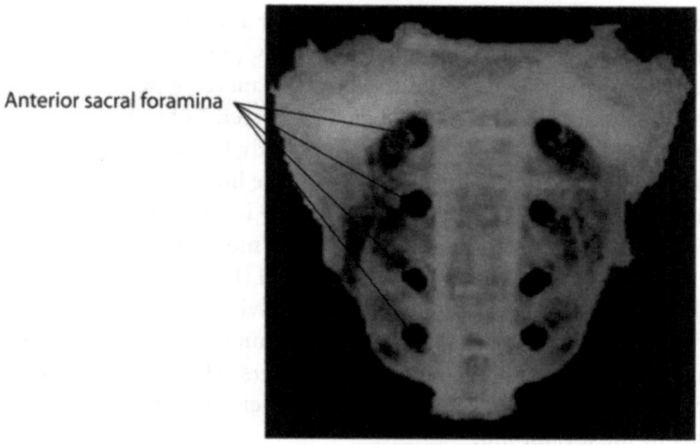

FIG. 4. Pelvic surface of the sacrum. Three-dimensional computerized axial tomography (CAT) reconstruction image using volume rendering

fasciae. The levator ani muscle is composed of the puborectalis muscle, the pubococcygeus muscle, and the iliococcygeus muscle.

Striated muscle exhibits a medium-intensity signal in T1-weighted MR images, and a decrease in signal intensity in T2-weighted images (Hricak and Carrington 1991).

The levator ani muscle (Fig. 1c,d,i,j,l,p) originates from the long linear region on the internal surface of the pelvic wall. The muscle begins on the posterior surface of the body of the pubis, and terminates at the ischial spine.

The anterior portion of the pubococcygeus muscle supports the urethra, the prostate in the male (levator prostate muscle), and the vagina in the female (pubovaginalis muscle).

The right and left pubococcygeus muscles unite in the midline region between the tip of the coccyx and the anorectal junction. The right and left iliococcygeus muscles also unite. The puborectalis muscle forms a muscular loop around the anorectal junction, and is called the anorectal sling.

The coccygeus muscle is posterosuperior to the levator ani. It arises from the pelvic surface and the tip of the ischial spine, and is attached to the lateral margin of the coccyx and fifth sacral vertebra. It supports the posterior part of the pelvic floor.

The perineum can be divided into the urogenital triangle (the anterior part) and the anal triangle (the posterior part). The muscles and fasciae of the urogenital triangle provide additional anterior pelvic outlet support where the levator musculature is relatively deficient (Klutke and Siegel 1995). The muscles and fasciae of the anal triangle are bounded behind by the tip of the coccyx, and on each side by the ischial tuberosity and sacrotuberous ligament. The urogenital triangle is bounded in front by the pubic arch, and laterally by the ischial tuberosities. The urogenital diaphragm (Fig. 1m) is in the urogenital triangle below the pelvic diaphragm. It is a thin, membranous muscular structure between the right and left pubic arches. It is mainly formed by the deep transverse perineus muscles and their fasciae. The perineal body

(Fig. 1b,i) divides the perineal muscles into anterior and posterior muscles. The anterior perineal muscles include the bulbospongiosus (Fig. 1b,i,m,n), the ischiocavernosus (Fig. 1b,i,m), and the deep and superficial transverse perineus (Fig. 1b,i). The posterior perineal muscle is the external anal sphincter. Not only do the anterior and posterior perineal muscles attach to the perineal body, but they also attach to the puborectalis muscle. The perineal body is similar to the hub of a wheel into which these various muscles, which provide pelvic support, are inserted like spokes (Klutke and Siegel 1995). Thus, the perineal body is one of the most important structures of the perineum, and is situated anterior to the anal canal (Fig. 1b,i).

The anal canal (Fig. 1b,i) is located below the pelvic floor. It descends between the anorectal ligament and the perineal body, and terminates at the anus. The anal canal walls are surrounded by a complex tube of sphincters. The associated muscular components are the internal and external anal sphincters, and the puborectalis muscle, which is part of the levator ani.

The ischiorectal fossa (Fig. 1c,j) is situated lateral to the rectum and anal canal, and medial to the internal obturator muscles and ischial tuberosity. It is filled with adipose tissue and covered by the obturator and levator ani fasciae. Anteriorly, the fossa is partly bounded by the posterior aspect of the muscles of the urogenital triangle. However, the ischiorectal fossa is prolonged above them as a narrow recess, sometimes reaching as far as the retropubic space (Williams et al. 1995). The axial and coronal planes, in which the levator ani muscles are routinely identified, are the optimal planes for imaging the ischiorectal fossa. The levator ani muscles constitute the most important anatomic and surgical landmark of this region (Llauger et al. 1998).

The pubis (Figs. 1c–e,j,p–r, 5) consists of a body and superior and inferior rami. The ischium (Fig. 1b–e,i,j,l,o) consists of a body and a ramus. The right and left bodies of the pubis are connected to each other at the pubic symphysis. The superior ramus of the pubis extends laterally from the upper part of the body and communicates with the acetabulum. The inferior ramus of the pubis is continuous with the ischial ramus, which is the inferior part of the ischium. The body of the ischium extends superiorly to form the inferoposterior portion of the acetabulum. The ischial tuberosity (Fig. 1c,o) is a large roughened area situated at the posteroinferior part of the ischium. The sacrotuberous ligament (Fig. 6) is attached distally to the ischial tuberosity, and fans out to the ischial ramus. The ischial spine (Fig. 1e) separates the greater and lesser sciatic notches. The sacrospinous ligament (Fig. 6) is attached to the ischial spine. The obturator foramen is located between the pubis and the ischium.

Ligaments of the Sacroiliac Joint

The sacrum and the ilium are held together by the anterior (ventral) sacroiliac ligament, the interosseous sacroiliac ligament, and the posterior (dorsal) sacroiliac ligament.

The anterior sacroiliac ligament is a thin structure traversing the sacroiliac joint anteriorly. It cannot be separated from the anterior joint capsule by imaging studies, but MR images show the anterior capsular complex as a hypointense, linear or minimally curved structure (Jaovisidha et al. 1996).

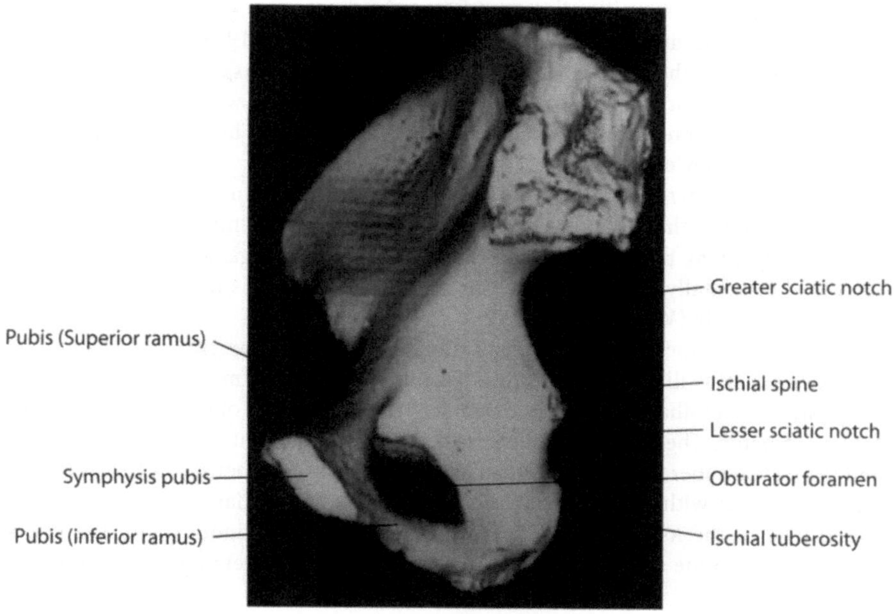

FIG. 5. Anteromedial surface of the right hip bone, showing the pubis and ischium. Three-dimensional CAT reconstruction image using shaped surface display

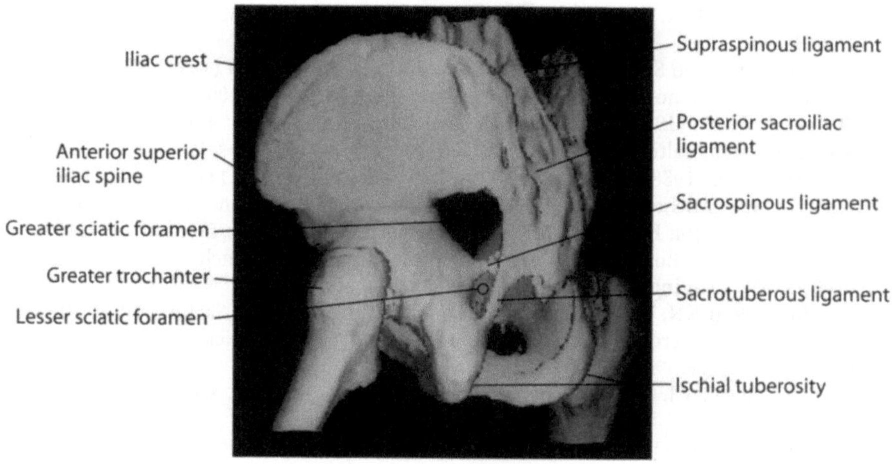

FIG. 6. Left posterolateral view of the ligaments of the sacroiliac joint. Three-dimensional reconstruction image using shaped surface display

The interosseous sacroiliac ligament forms the major connection to the irregular space posterosuperior to the sacroiliac joint (Williams et al. 1995). MR imaging can clearly distinguish the synovial and ligamentous compartments of the sacroiliac joint. The ligamentous portion of the joint contains adipose tissue, with focal areas of low signal intensity representing loose connective tissue and the interosseous sacroiliac ligament (Murphey et al. 1991).

The posterior sacroiliac ligament (Fig. 6) lies over the interosseous ligament, with the dorsal rami of the sacral spinal nerves and vessels intervening. The short posterior iliac ligament represents the deeper portion of the ligament, with its fibers directed horizontally. The long posterior sacroiliac ligament is more superficial and oriented vertically (Williams et al. 1995).

On the cranial side, the long posterior (dorsal) sacroiliac ligament is attached to the posterior superior iliac spine and the adjacent part of the ilium. On the caudal side, the posterior sacroiliac ligament is attached to the lateral crest of the third and fourth sacral segments. The main part of the sacrotuberous ligament connects the sacrum and the ischial tuberosity (Vleeming et al. 1996). The sacrotuberous ligament is partially combined with the posterior sacroiliac ligament (Williams et al. 1995). The lateral part of the long posterior sacroiliac ligament is continuous with the fibers passing between the ischial tuberosity and the iliac bone (Vleeming et al. 1996).

References

Blake LC, Robertson WD, Hayes CE (1996) Sacral plexus: optimal imaging planes for MR assessment. Radiology 199:767–772

Dooms GC, Hricak H, Tscholakoff D (1986) Adnexal structures: MR imaging. Radiology 158:639–646

Gierada DS, Erickson SJ, Haughton VM, Estkowski LD, Nowicki BH (1993) MR imaging of the sacral plexus: normal findings. Am J Roentgenol 160:1059–1065

Hall-Craggs ECB (1985) Anatomy as the basis for clinical medicine. Urban & Schwarzenberg, Baltimore, Munich, pp 326–386

Heiken JP, Lee JK (1988) MR imaging of the pelvis. Radiology 166:11–16

Hricak H (1986) MRI of the female pelvis: a review. Am J Roentgenol 146:1115–1122

Hricak H, Carrington BM (1991) MRI of the pelvis. Martin Dunitz, London, pp 43–91

Hricak H, Secaf E, Buckley DW, Brown JJ, Tanagho EA, McAninch JW (1991) Female urethra: MR imaging. Radiology 178:527–535

Jaovisidha S, Ryu KN, De Maeseneer M, Haghighi P, Goodwin D, Sartoris DJ, Resnick D (1996) Ventral sacroiliac ligament. Anatomic and pathologic considerations. Invest Radiol 31:532–541

Klutke CG, Siegel CL (1995) Functional female pelvic anatomy. Urol Clin North Am 22:487–498

Lanzieri CF, Hilal SK (1984) Computed tomography of the sacral plexus and sciatic nerve in the greater sciatic foramen. Am J Roentgenol 143:165–168

Llauger J, Palmer J, Perez C, Monill J, Ribe J, Moreno A (1998) The normal and pathologic ischiorectal fossa at CT and MR imaging. Radiographics 18:61–82

Murphey MD, Wetzel LH, Bramble JM, Levine E, Simpson KM, Lindsley HB (1991) Sacroiliitis: MR imaging findings. Radiology 180:239–244

Pearl RK, Monsen H, Abcarian H (1986) Surgical anatomy of the pelvic autonomic nerves. A practical approach. Am Surg 52:236–237

Secaf E, Nuruddin RN, Hricak H, McClure RD, Demas B (1991) MR imaging of the seminal vesicles. Am J Roentgenol 156:989–994

Sommer FG, McNeal JE, Carrol CL (1986) MR depiction of the zonal anatomy of the prostate at 1.5 T. J Comput Assist Tomogr 10:983–989
Togashi K (1993) MRI of the female pelvis. Igaku-Shoin, Tokyo, pp 29–68
Vleeming A, Pool-Goudzwaard AL, Hammudoghlu D, Stoeckart R, Snijders CJ, Mens JM (1996) The function of the long dorsal sacroiliac ligament: its implication for understanding low back pain. Spine 21:556–562
Williams PL, Bannister LH, Collins P, Dyson M, Dyson M, Dussek JE, Ferguson MWJ (eds) (1995) Gray's anatomy: the anatomical basis of medicine and surgery. Churchill Livingstone, New York, pp 528–529, 674–677, 832

Imaging Examinations of Tumors

Tetsuo Hotta

Summary. Imaging examinations must be done prior to any kind of surgical intervention, including biopsy. Many kinds of imaging examination are now available, but they are not equally important in relation to the tumor surgery. A three-dimensional image of the location of a bone tumor is best obtained by a computed axial tomography (CAT) scan. For soft-tissue tumors, a magnetic resonance (MR) image is the best diagnostic tool. Angiography is still necessary before pelvic surgery.

Key words. Computed axial tomography, Magnetic resonance imaging, Angiography, Pyelography, Sacrectomy

Introduction

Prior to the 1970s, only standard X-ray assessment and angiography were available for preoperative planning of pelvic tumor surgery. Even in the early stages of limb salvage surgery, computerized axial tomography (CAT) scans were not routinely performed. We experienced many cases of inadequate resection or major complications due mainly to the lack of adequate preoperative imaging information. Recently, however, many powerful imaging tools have become available. This is perhaps the single most important reason for recent improvements in pelvic tumor surgery. Routine imaging examinations for preoperative planning should include X-ray, CAT scan, magnetic resonance (MR) imaging, and angiography.

Examination

A CAT scan is superior to MR imaging for planning pelvic tumor surgery. A three-dimensional CAT scan is the most powerful tool currently available. The space resolution of a CAT scan is better than that of an MR image. MR imaging frequently exaggerates the margin of the tumor, and makes it unclear. MR imaging is effective in detecting the intramedullary extent of a tumor, and its intramuscular invasion. Three-dimensional CAT scans provide a great deal of information which is helpful for planning the surgery using paper templates. Three-dimensional angiography is also available by CAT scan. Vascular dissection is easier with preoperative information from a three-dimensional CAT scan. Imaging also allows the preoperative preparation of vascular reconstructions.

A key point in pelvic tumor surgery is thought to be the clearance of the greater sciatic notch. The sacroiliac joint can be osteotomized if the notch is widely exposed. The success of a sacrectomy and internal hemipelvectomy depend upon this point. Imaging should mainly be used to evaluate the clearance of the greater sciatic notch.

Angiography has not been very useful in tumor surgery on the extremities, but remains very important in pelvic tumor surgery. The invasion and involvement of the external and internal iliac arteries must be carefully assessed. In particular, the internal iliac artery and its branches should be studied in detail. Embolization is performed in the examination, if necessary.

If the tumor is close to the promontory of the sacrum, drip infusion pyelography is necessary to assess the involvement of the ureter.

After all essential imaging examinations have been performed, the surgery can be planned using paper templates, and then reproduced in the operating room.

Chapter 2
Incidence and Histological Classification

Incidence and Histological Classification of Pelvic Tumors

Akira Ogose

Summary. The most common locations and histological classifications of primary pelvic tumors in 130 patients were analyzed. Chondrosarcoma is the most common tumor in the pelvis.

Key words. Chondrosarcoma, Malignant fibrous histiocytoma

One hundred and thirty patients with pelvic tumors underwent surgical treatment in Niigata University Hospital from 1969 to 1999. The specific anatomic locations and the numbers of cases of each are summarized in Table 1. Tumors involving the ilium and pelvic soft tissues each accounted for approximately one-third of the total number of cases. The most commonly encountered tumors at our institution were metastatic tumors. Surgical treatment for metastatic tumors is very difficult in most cases because the metastasis tends to be multiple and extensive, and the general condition of the patient is usually poor. Associated malignant lymphoma and myeloma often develop in the pelvis.

Table 1. Location of pelvic tumors

Location	No. of cases
Ilium	43
Pubis	8
Ischium	9
Sacrum	31
Soft tissue	39
Total	130

Table 2. Tumors of the ilium

Tumor type	No. of cases
Chondrosarcoma	10
Bone cyst	6
Ewing's sarcoma	5
Osteosarcoma	4
Histiocytosis X	4
Giant cell tumor	2
Fibrous dysplasia	2
Aneurysmal bone cyst	2
Exostosis	2
Malignant fibrous histiocytoma	2
Angiosarcoma	1
Fibrosarcoma	1
Lymphoma	1
Myositis ossificans	1
Total	43

TABLE 3. Tumors of the pubis

Tumor type	No. of cases
Chondrosarcoma	4
Osteosarcoma	1
Bone cyst	1
Ewing's sarcoma	1
Exostosis	1
Total	8

TABLE 4. Tumors of the ischium

Tumor type	No. of cases
Aneurysmal bone cyst	3
Exostosis	2
Osteosarcoma	1
Histiocytosis X	1
Fibrous dysplasia	1
Hemangioma	1
Total	9

TABLE 5. Tumors of the sacrum

Tumor type	No. of cases
Chordoma	8
Giant cell tumor	7
Schwannoma	4
Chondrosarcoma	2
Osteosarcoma	1
Fibrosarcoma	1
Malignant fibrous histiocytoma	1
Angiosarcoma	1
Lymphoma	1
Desmoplastic fibroma	1
Fibrous dysplasia	1
Hemangioma	1
Teratoma	1
Lipoma	1
Total	31

TABLE 6. Tumors of the soft tissue around the pelvis

Tumor type	No. of cases
Malignant fibrous histiocytoma	7
Liposarcoma	5
Hemangioma	5
Malignant peripheral nerve sheath	4
Lipoma	3
Schwannoma	3
Neurofibroma	3
Fibrosarcoma	3
Epidermal cyst	2
Ewing's sarcoma	1
Synovial sarcoma	1
Desmoid tumor	1
Myxoma	1
Total	39

The most common type of primary bone tumor encountered in the ilium was a chondrosarcoma, which accounted for nearly one-quarter of the tumors of the ilium at our institution (Table 2). Bone cyst, Ewing's sarcoma, osteosarcoma, and histiocytosis X also occurred in the ilium, with each type representing approximately 10% of the tumors of the ilium.

A chondrosarcoma was the most common tumor in the pubis, accounting for one-half of the tumors of the pubis at our institution (Table 3).

An aneurysmal bone cyst was the most commonly occurring tumor in the ischium, representing one-third of the tumors of the ischium (Table 4).

A chordoma and giant cell tumor were the most common primary bone tumors found in the sacrum, each accounting for nearly one-quarter of the tumors of the sacrum at our institution (Table 5). In addition, a schwannoma and chondrosarcoma should also be considered in the differential diagnosis of sacral tumors.

The most common soft tissue tumors in the pelvis were malignant fibrous histiocytoma, liposarcoma, hemangioma, and malignant peripheral nerve sheath tumor (Table 6). Lipoma, schwannoma, neurofibroma, and fibrosarcoma also occurred.

Chapter 3
Biopsy

Efficacy of Aspiration Cytology and a Practical Method of Open Biopsy

Tetsuo Hotta

Summary. Aspiration biopsy cytology (ABC) is recommended for pelvic tumors to reduce the risk of tumor contamination and complications such as massive bleeding. ABC is available not only for soft tissue tumors, but also for bone tumors. The accuracy rate of ABC for bone tumors is over 90% in our data. If there is a discrepancy between the cytological diagnosis and imaging, then open biopsy is necessary. An open biopsy of acetabular lesions is more difficult than for other lesions because of the anatomy of the region. Of several possible approaches for acetabular lesions, that involving the detachment of the gluteal muscle from the ilium may be the best option if it is strongly suspected that the tumor is malignant.

Key words. Aspiration cytology, Open biopsy, Complications, Timing, Approach

Introduction

In the 1970s, a hindquarter amputation was the only option for the surgical removal of a malignant pelvic tumor. An open biopsy could be performed with relative ease without being disadvantageous to ablative surgery. However, limb-sparing surgery to remove malignant pelvic tumors is now available in many cases. Because of this, a biopsy must not only be diagnostic, but must also be carefully performed so that successful limb-salvage surgery can be achieved.

Obtaining a biopsy of a pelvic tumor is difficult because of the anatomy of the pelvis. The tumor is usually deeply seated and surrounded by vital tissues and organs. If the tumor is malignant, an open biopsy often leads to complications such the sciatic nerve or a major artery becoming contaminated with tumor tissue. For example, the sciatic nerve may become contaminated with tumor tissue when obtaining a biopsy of a liquefied tumor such as a myxoid chondrosarcoma using a posterior ischial approach. Sparing the nerve increases the risk of local recurrence. However, it is also possible that the sciatic nerve may be unnecessarily sacrificed. In some cases, a wide margin cannot be achieved after open biopsy because of the extensive bleeding.

The skin incision for a biopsy should be carefully considered. If an inadequate skin incision is made, an ideal approach for tumor removal can rarely be achieved. In many cases, adequate skin coverage of the wound is very difficult to obtain, even in untreated cases, because the circulation in the flap is easily disturbed by massive muscle resection. If the skin incision for a biopsy is made in the center of the buttock, a gluteal flap can no longer be used, and a local flap would be required. The skin incision must be made following the ilioinguinal and posterior iliac approaches.

We prefer to use fine-needle aspiration biopsy cytology in order to avoid the significant disadvantages associated with an open biopsy. We have achieved a high rate of diagnostic accuracy, even in the cytology of bone tumors of the extremities (Hotta et al. 1996). Of course, the cooperation of a trained pathologist is essential to ensure that the cytological diagnosis is reliably diagnostic. If an accurate aspiration of the lesion is achieved, a cytological diagnosis of pelvic bone and soft tissue tumors can accurate and reliable. We have developed a fine-needle aspiration system with a special hole-in-one device for penetrating the hard cortex or a sclerosing bone tumor. Our method of fine-needle aspiration cytology is explained below. The limitations of cytological diagnoses and the indications for open biopsy are also discussed.

Fine-Needle Aspiration Biopsy Cytology (ABC)

Fine-needle aspiration biopsy cytology (ABC) is a powerful diagnostic tool, especially in the case of pelvic tumors. ABC is a safe, easy, and time-saving method of histological diagnosis. It is also less invasive and more repeatable than other methods. In adult patients, all trials are performed under local anesthesia. Twenty-one pelvic bone tumors and 12 soft tissue tumors were aspirated, and cytological diagnoses were made. The sensitivity of the diagnosis of malignancy was 93%, and the specificity was 90%. The total accuracy rate was 91%. Histological diagnoses of tumors such as a chondrosarcoma or osteosarcoma were successfully made in 50% of the total number of aspirations. An Enneking's Stage II B (high-grade) tumor was easily aspirated from an extraosseous lesion. We developed a hole-in-one cannulated drill system for a fine needle. It is guided by a 1.5-mm-diameter Kirschner wire. When it is confirmed by an image intensifier or computerized axial tomography (CAT) scan that the tip of the Kirschner wire is positioned in the bone tumor, a fragile fine needle can be introduced easily and safely into the tumor. An intraosseous chondrosarcoma was also successfully aspirated by this method. Two cases of chordoma involving the sacrum were diagnosed by the CAT-guided approach. There were no major or minor complications. The needle tract was resected whenever possible. However, this was not done in about half of all the bone and soft tissue tumor cases. When ABC was performed with an 18-gauge needle, no local recurrence of the tumor was observed from the tract. Nonetheless, the needle tract should be made on the line of surgery, and should be resected if possible. However, if a fine-needle tract cannot be resected, the tumor cells are not likely to contaminate the tract. Therefore, a fine-needle tract may remain unresected, but it is best to make the tract as far as possible from the major vessels and nerves.

Cancer metastasis is the best indication for cytology. Hemorrhagic metastases such as a renal cell carcinoma, thyroid carcinoma, or hepatoma are suitable candidates. These lesions were safely aspirated and accurately diagnosed by ABC in our outpatient clinic.

Low-grade tumors such as a low-grade osteosarcoma, or purely sclerotic lesions such as in Paget's disease, may not be reliably diagnosed by ABC alone. Accurate cytological diagnoses of cystic lesions such as a unicameral bone cyst or an aneurysmal bone cyst are also difficult. Cystic changes in a malignant tumor do not provide representative cells in many cases. Such situations represent a limitation or contraindication of the ABC method. We have made diagnoses of secondary chondrosarcomas arising from exostoses in the pelvis by using imaging techniques only, i.e., a standard X-ray, magnetic resonance imaging, or a CAT scan. These cases were treated surgically without biopsy, and were found to be chondrosarcomas, and not exostoses.

Open Biopsy

If there is a discrepancy between the cytological diagnosis and imaging, then an open biopsy is necessary. The skin incision for an open biopsy should be made on the line of the wide excision surgery, as mentioned previously. Intraosseous acetabular lesions and ischial lesions are the most difficult lesions for open biopsy.

Three approaches are available for an acetabular tumor. The first is the Smith–Peterson approach. This has a high degree of risk of contamination of the femoral nerve and vessels. The second approach is the direct transmuscular (gluteus medius) approach. If the tumor is malignant, this approach requires resection of the gluteus medius muscle. In addition, when this approach is used, the lesion is usually found to be very deep-seated. The third approach provides a wider exposure by detaching the gluteus muscle from the ilium. This approach is the most invasive, but a portion of the hip abductors can be preserved even if the lesion is malignant. This approach also has the advantage that the skin incision can be made on the line of the wide resection. Generally, the approach involving the detachment of the muscle from the ilium may be the best option if it is strongly suspected that the tumor is malignant.

Two approaches are possible for an ischial tumor. The first is the posterior ischial approach, and the second is the direct approach from the ischial tubercle. In the former approach, the sciatic nerve is almost always exposed and contaminated with malignant cells. The latter approach has a high risk of infection, and careful sanitary care is necessary after a biopsy. However, the latter approach is recommended.

Key Points of an Open Biopsy

The cooperation of a trained musculoskeletal tumor pathologist is essential for an accurate histological diagnosis. However, a surgeon should obtain the representative specimen. A sufficient amount of specimen is necessary. The biopsy must be cleanly harvested, not crushed by a clamp, and quickly fixed. If the lesion is cartilaginous, a block specimen containing the cortex should be harvested. In a low-grade chondrosarcoma, the only evidence of malignancy is the permeation of the tumor tissue into the preexisting trabeculae, and the invasion of the cortex by the tumor. These features cannot be confirmed from biopsy tissue harvested piecemeal.

Bleeding must be completely controlled by electrocoagulation or ligature. Fenestration of the cortex should be packed with bone cement. Fascia or muscle which had been lying over the tumor must be tightly sutured. Suction drains should not be inserted, since the tract may become contaminated after removal of the drain.

Reference

Hotta T, Emura I, Saito H, Inoue Y, Ogose A, Yamamura S (1996) Fine-needle aspiration cytology of bone and soft-tissue tumors. Orthop Trans 20:213

Chapter 4
Preparation

Preparation, Intraoperative Care, and Postoperative Treatment

Tetsuro Morita

Summary. The most important preoperative preparation task is the cleaning of the patient's bowel. A combination of an enema and cathartics is recommended. Situations with expected blood loss without complications are listed according to the individual procedures. Intraoperative care is essential to avoid compression sores and nerve palsy. The positioning check points are described in this chapter. The timetable for the rehabilitation program is also explained.

Key words. Bowel cleaning, Urogenital sterilization, Blood loss, Compression sores, Rehabilitation

Introduction

Patients with malignant pelvic tumors usually require over 10h operative time, and a blood transfusion of over one liter. A preoperative evaluation of the medical status of the patient is very important. A determination of the presence of any metabolic disease, and an assessment of cardiovascular and respiratory function should be carried out. If a patient's medical condition is thought to represent a high risk factor for major surgery, radiation-assisted reduction surgery or radiation therapy may be recommended. Inadequate reduction surgery almost always results in local recurrence and subsequent death. If a colostomy or urinary diversion is thought to be necessary, there must be preoperative consultation with general surgeons and urologists, and the combined surgical team must be assembled. Our team has no definite opinion about the need for a prophylactic colostomy, but a colostomy should probably not be done if at all possible.

Preparation

The most important preoperative preparatory task is cleaning the patient's bowel. If the bowel is not cleaned before surgery, wide exposure of the intrapelvic cavity cannot be obtained. We prefer a combination of an enema and cathartics. Our routine is to give the patient a clear liquid diet for 2 days, followed by a strong laxative or cathartics administrated 24h before surgery. In addition, an enema is administered early in the morning of the day of surgery. A more formal method of bowel preparation is

TABLE 1. Expected blood loss during pelvic surgery

Type of resection	Intraoperative blood loss (ml)	Postoperative bleeding (ml)
Conventional hemipelvectomy	800–3500	200–600
Internal hemipelvectomy	1500–5000	200–800
Resection of type I	400–2000	100–200
Resection of type II		
Prosthesis	1500–3000	200–400
Arthrodesis	2000–4000	300–600
Resection of type III	400–2000	100–300
Sacral amputation	800–2000	100–200
Total sacrectomy	3000–6000	400–1000

required if there is a risk that the bowel will be operated on during surgery. If a longer operative time is anticipated, several days' of preoperative intravenous hyperalimentation is effective both for cleaning the bowel and for maintaining the patient's physical strength. A large retroperitoneal tumor may involve the ureter, colon, or rectum. In such cases, urinary diversion, nephrectomy, or a colostomy is necessary during surgery, or prior to pelvic surgery. If it is suspected that the tumor is close to the ureter, ureteral catheterization may be necessary.

A urogenital fungus infection and endocervicitis of the uterus are serious risk factors for early infection. These septic conditions must be completely cleared up preoperatively. We have experienced an intractable enterococcus infection from endometritis.

A patient with a significant pelvic lesion requires from 6 to 20 h operative time and a massive blood transfusion, depending on the surgical stage, the histological diagnosis, and the experience of the surgical team. Stored autogenous blood reinfusion is effective only in limited cases. Sufficient blood for intraoperative and postoperative infusion should be prepared. When expecting a massive blood loss of over 2000 ml, fresh frozen plasma should also be prepared in order to avoid coagulopathies. Situations in which one would expect blood loss without complications are listed in Table 1. These, of course, are representative scenarios, and may be minimum quantities. More transfused blood may be needed, depending on the surgical stage, the histology, the experience of the surgeons, or the occurrence of unexpected vascular complications.

Intraoperative Care

The operative time required is usually longer than originally anticipated. The patient should be carefully positioned to avoid compression sores or nerve palsy. The head, neck, and all extremities should be carefully padded and positioned. In the lateral decubitus position, an auxiliary roll or some other type of pressure relief is recommended for the shoulder in contact with the table.

Blood loss should be carefully monitored by both the anesthesia and surgical teams. The patient often receives a blood transfusion late in the procedure because of unexpected massive bleeding. Early blood transfusion is recommended in order to avoid coagulopathies and circulatory disturbance.

Postoperative Management

The suction drain is left in place until there is less than 50 ml of drainage fluid over a 24-h period. Postoperative drainage usually seems to be greater in Japanese patients than in American patients. However, the drain should be removed within a week in order to avoid infection, even if the volume of drainage is greater than 50 ml.

In a case of hemipelvectomy, the patient is encouraged to get out of bed as soon as possible, usually within a few days after surgery. Young people can walk with crutches, but elderly patients require staged rehabilitation, progressing from standing on a tilt table to using a walker for ambulation. Most adults do not use a Canadian prosthesis for ambulating. Children and young adults may be able to use a prosthesis, and should be encouraged to do so.

Postoperative management of type I (iliac) and type III (ischiopubic) resections is almost the same as for a hemipelvectomy, because patients with these resections usually do not require any reconstruction (Enneking and Dunham 1978; Hotta 2000; O'Connor and Sim 1989; Steel 1978).

A type II (acetabular) resection usually requires reconstruction of the hip joint. Total hip arthroplasty (THA) and hip arthrodesis are the major reconstruction procedures currently used. Prophylactic systemic intravenous antibiotics are routinely used for 1 week after surgery. It is often necessary to accompany THA with pelvic reconstruction using customized prostheses, methylmethacrylate, or allograft. Patients who have had a THA reconstruction are managed in the same way as any other patients with a THA. Patients with a reconstruction using bone cement are encouraged to move as soon as possible. If a soft tissue repair has been performed, immobilization in bed may be necessary for at least 3 weeks. The patient is allowed to sit up after 1 week. If the hip arthroplasty is unstable, a hip spica cast is recommended for 8 weeks. After the cast is removed, the patient is encouraged to perform isometric muscle-power exercises. The hip joint is gradually flexed, and the patient is allowed to sit up 3 weeks after the removal of the cast. Soft tissue contracture prevents dislocation of the hip joint after 3 months. If a bone graft or allograft has been used, the patient is immobilized in bed for 4 weeks. The hip joint is gradually flexed, and the patient is then allowed to sit up during the next 2 weeks. Standing exercises on the unaffected limb are begun on a tilt table, and continued for 2 weeks. Non-weight-bearing gait follows. Partial weight-bearing is allowed, depending upon evidence of a union. This typically requires at least 3–6 months.

Patients who have undergone arthrodesis are typically placed in a hip spica cast because the internal fixation with this procedure is usually less than optimal. Such patients should be encouraged to perform standing exercises, since these can be performed even in a hip spica cast.

References

Enneking WF, Dunham WK (1978) Resection and reconstruction for primary neoplasms involving the innominate bone. J Bone Joint Surg Am 60:731–746

Hotta T (2000) Ischiopubic bone tumors. Proceedings of the 3rd Meeting of the Asia Pacific Musculoskeletal Tumor Society, Hong Kong, p 86

O'Connor MI, Sim FH (1989) Salvage of the limb in the treatment of malignant pelvic tumors. J Bone Joint Surg Am 71:481–494
Steel HH (1978) Partial or complete resection of the hemipelvis. An alternative to hindquarter amputation for periacetabular chondrosarcoma of the pelvis. J Bone Joint Surg Am 60:719–730

Chapter 5
Approach

Systemic Surgical Approach for the Pelvis

Tetsuo Hotta

Summary. The surgical approach for the individual parts of the pelvis is described in detail. The posterior sacral and anterior sacral (Stener's) approaches are used for the sacrum. The ilioinguinal and posterior iliac approaches are used for the ilium. The transperineal and posterior ischial aproaches are used for the ischiopubic bone. The procedures of sacral amputation, total sacrectomy, and internal hemipelvectomy are also explained, with abundant illustrations.

Key words. Posterior sacral approach, Anterior extraperitoneal approach, Ilioinguinal approach, Sacral amputation, Internal hemipelvectomy

Sacrum

Posterior Sacral Approach

The posterior sacral approach is used in two situations. One application is in combination with an anterior approach for a total sacrectomy. The other application is when performing a sacral amputation below the level of S2. S2 cannot be resected through a posterior approach only, but a sacral amputation between S2 and S3 can be performed with this approach. This procedure may be indicated for a small chordoma.

Surgical Procedure: Sacral Amputation (Samson et al. 1993; Waisman et al. 1997)

When performing a sacral amputation, a reverse Y-shaped skin incision is made at the midline of the sacrum (Fig. 1). This incision allows easy exposure of the lateral margin of the sacrum, the sacrotuberous ligament, and the sacrospinous ligament. These ligaments are very thick and tight, and should be transected first (Fig. 2). The sciatic notch must be widely exposed in order to identify the sciatic nerve, the piriformis muscle, the superior gluteal artery, and the inferior gluteal artery. The spinal canal is exposed at the intended amputation level by performing a laminectomy, and the nerve roots are ligated and cut. If possible, the S2 nerve root on one side of the sacrum should be preserved in order to maintain vesicorectal function. Both S2 nerve roots are identified in the spinal canal, and the neural foramen is identified through a wider laminectomy. The osteotomy line of the sacrum is marked on the posterior

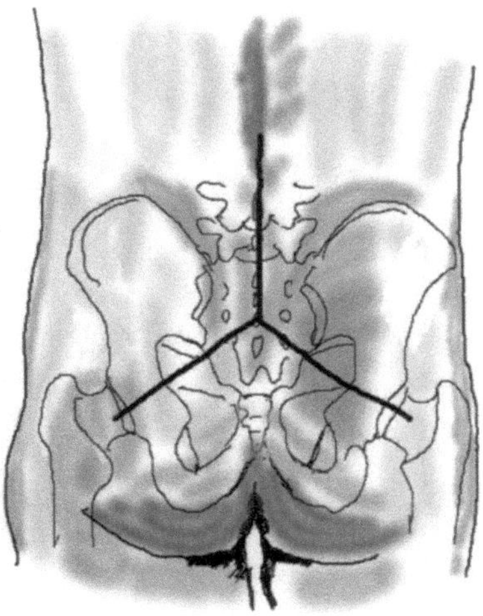

FIG. 1. Posterior sacral approach. This particular posterior sacral approach is used for a sacral amputation and total sacrectomy. The upper half of the reverse Y-shaped skin incision is made straight on the spinous processes. The point of bifurcation is located on the level of the greater sciatic notch or two fingers breadth below, and the branch of reverse Y runs toward the greater trochanter of the femur

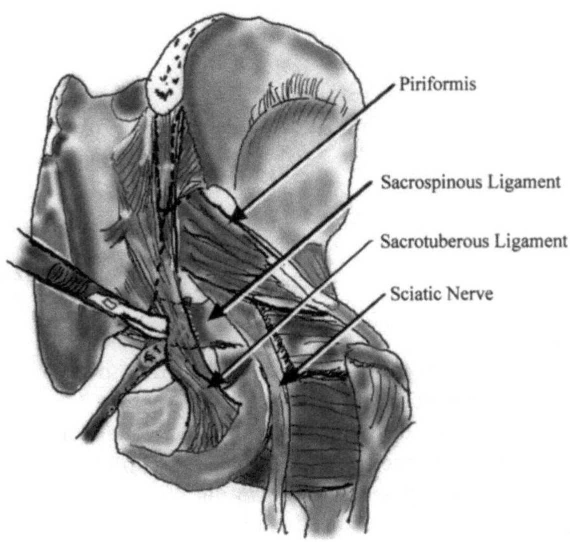

FIG. 2. Tight ligaments between the sacrum and the ischium. These ligaments should be cut first. Great care must be taken to identify and protect the sciatic nerve. It usually locates laterally to the ligaments

wall. A gutter is made on the osteotomy line using Luel forceps or a high-speed burr (Fig. 3).

The anterior aspect of the sacrum can be exposed by gradual blunt dissection. The anterior wall of the osteotomy line can be resected, piece-by-piece, using a Kerrison rongeur as illustrated in Fig. 3. This maneuver should be carefully performed after anterior blunt dissection. It is very difficult to perform the osteotomy through the midline of the sacrum since the center of the sacral body is very thick. However, if the lateral gutter on both sides of the sacrum is sufficiently wide, a sponge or retractor can be safely introduced beneath the anterior sacral wall, as illustrated in Fig. 4.

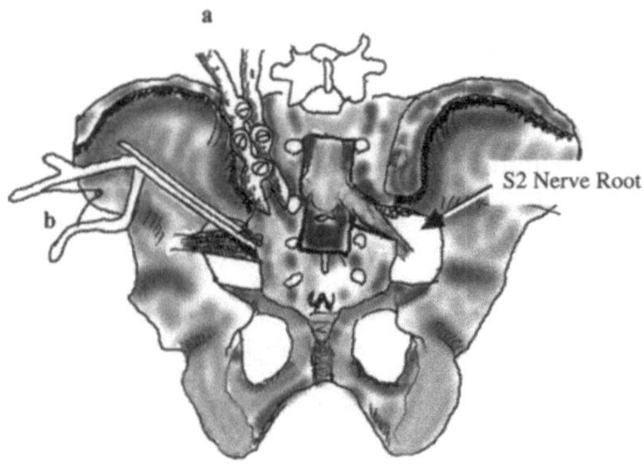

FIG. 3. Lateral gutter of the amputation level. A posterior gutter is made with Luel forceps. An anterior gutter is made piece by piece with a Kerrison rongeur. Laminectomy is made on the S1 and S2 level. The dural tube is already ligated and transected. A wide lateral gutter is made in the right side, and the right S2 nerve root is fully exposed

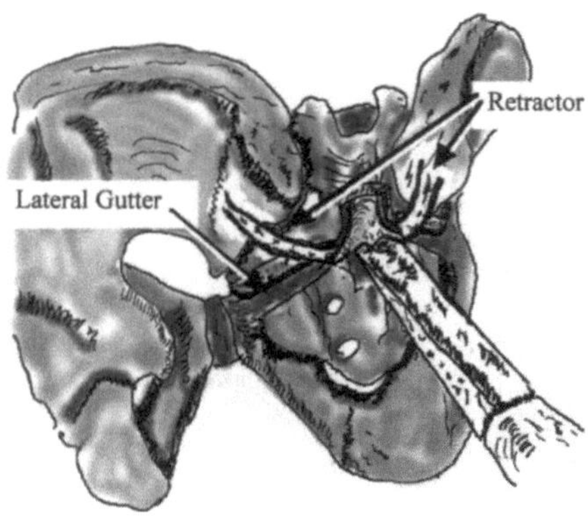

FIG. 4. Final osteotomy of the sacral body. Two retractors are introduced between the body and the presacral soft tissue to protect the major vessels and the rectum. The osteotomy is performed with an osteotome

The midportion of the sacrum can then be osteotomized with an osteotome. The sacral osteotomy is then completed.

Dissection of the tumor should be made from the proximal to the distal end. Soft tissues positioned between the rectum and the sacrum at the osteotomy level should be carefully dissected by elevating the cut stump of the sacrum (Fig. 5). The stump should be reflected distally, and the rectum bluntly dissected. There is typically some soft tissue between the sacrum and the rectum, and the rectum can be freed from the tumor. The branches of the internal iliac artery and vein are too deeply located to be dealt with in the anterior approach. However, they are easily managed in this particular situation. The sacral amputation is then completed (Fig. 6).

A wide dead space remains, but no special reconstruction procedure is necessary. In most cases, the skin flaps can be directly sutured. Patients with a sacral amputation have sometimes complained of difficulty with the evacuation of stools because the rectum had become unstable in the dead space. Recent attempts have been made to form a counter wall on the sacral defect using a marlex mesh sheet (Fig. 7), but the outcome of this type of procedure is not yet known. If the dead space is too large to avoid infection, it should be packed with antibiotic-impregnated cement beads (Ozaki et al. 1997). The beads should be removed several months later.

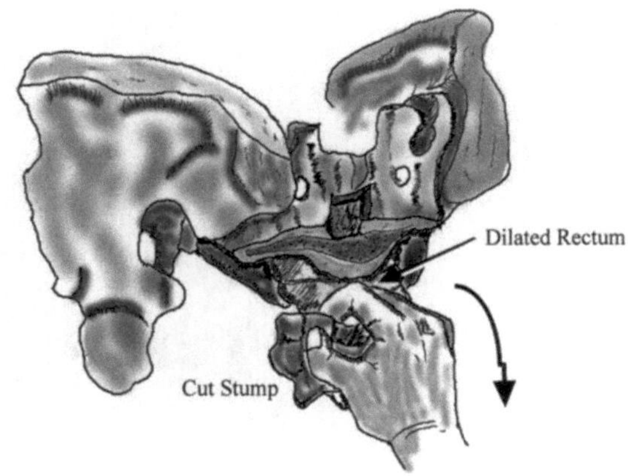

FIG. 5. Presacral dissection. The cut stump of the sacrum is elevated, and a blunt dissection is made between the sacrum and the rectum. There is typically some soft tissue between the sacrum and the rectum

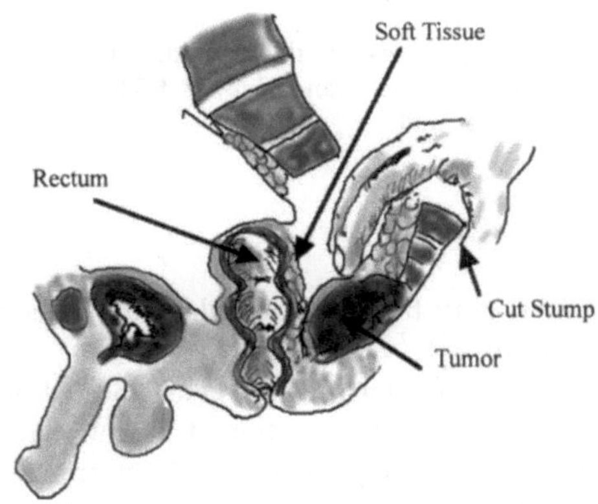

FIG. 6. Completed sacral amputation

Sacral amputation can be performed with a posterior approach. However, the following point should be carefully checked preoperatively. Adhesion between the rectum and the tumor should be assessed by imaging and digital anal examination. It is also useful to consult a general surgeon. If adhesion is suspected, a posterior approach is not indicated.

Anterior Extraperitoneal Sacral Approach

The purpose of an anterior approach is to expose the sacroiliac joint completely up to the greater sciatic notch, and to expose the upper vertebral osteotomy level, which may be the L5/S1 disc or any lumbar spinal body. The osteotomy should be completed with a posterior approach. The main purpose of the anterior approach is the exposure and protection of important structures.

Angiography should always be performed in order to answer three important questions.

1. Can the external iliac vessels be preserved? If not, replacement vessels must be prepared. An artificial artery usually works well, but an artificial vein does not. A

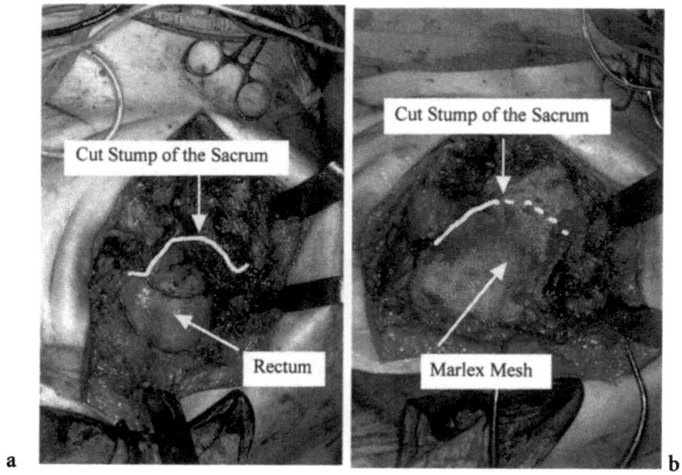

Fig. 7. Counter wall on the sacral defect. **a** The dilated rectum can be seen after sacral amputation between the S2 and S3 levels. **b** The defect is covered with marlex mesh sheet, which acts as a counter wall

venous graft from the contralateral greater saphenous vein can be used (Case 13 in Chap. 10).

2. Are the internal iliac vessels located on the tumor? If they are located beneath the tumor, complete ligation of the internal iliac artery is necessary in the first stage of the anterior approach. If both internal iliac arteries must be sacrificed, then total resection of the bladder, rectum, and uterus is necessary. This may be a contraindication for surgery. The internal iliac vein should be preserved until all dissection is completed, because massive bleeding with congestion may be encountered.

3. Are there any feeders? If there is a feeder, blood loss can be decreased by ligation or embolization.

Surgical Procedure

The bowel must always be emptied in the usual manner. The patient is placed in the supine position or the lithotomy position. A large U-shaped Stener's incision is made (Fig. 8) (Stener and Gunterberg 1978). The following maneuvers are explained in detail in the section on the ilioinguinal approach below (and see Figs. 15–18). The abdominal muscles are carefully transected, and the retroperitoneal space is widely exposed. The inguinal canal usually is not opened, and the spermatic cords are compressed distally. Both the inferior epigastric artery and vein must be ligated and severed. The external iliac vessels and ureter must then be identified. If necessary, a ureter catheter can be used to find the ureter, although it can usually be identified without catheterization. The ureter passes over the bifurcation of the external and internal arteries. However, if any previous surgery has been performed, a ureter catheter should be placed since adhesions make dissection of the ureter difficult.

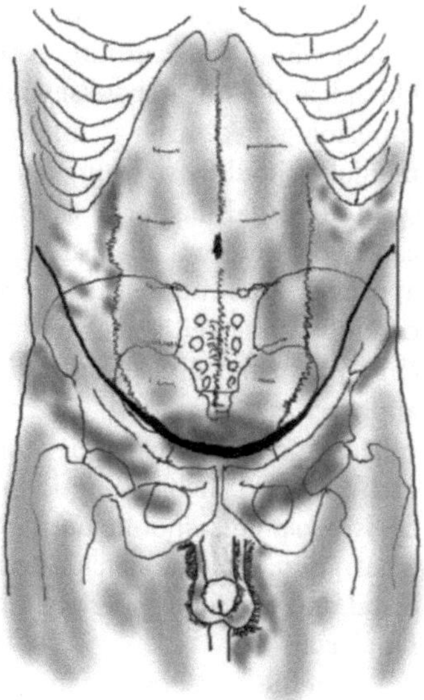

FIG. 8. Stener's anterior sacral approach. A large U-shaped skin incision is made. This is almost the same as the combined bilateral ilioinguinal approach

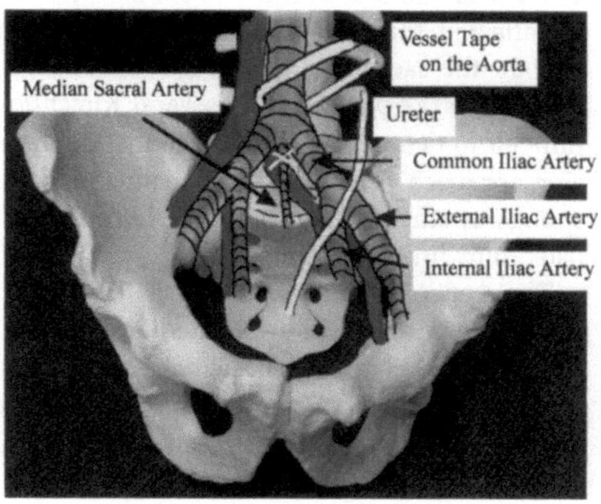

FIG. 9. View of the major vessels and the ureter. The aorta is isolated with vessel tape. The bifurcation of the abdominal aorta is usually located on the L4/5 spinal disc. The common iliac vessels, external iliac vessels, and internal iliac vessels are exposed. The ureter runs just on the bifurcation of the external and internal arteries. The median sacral artery is already ligated and severed

The external iliac vessels, internal iliac vessels, common iliac vessels, and abdominal aorta should then be exposed. The aorta can usually be exposed through this approach. The aorta is isolated with vessel tape. If necessary, bleeding can be controlled by temporarily clamping the aorta with a Fogarty clamp. The aorta can safely be clamped for up to 90 min at a time. The common iliac artery should also be isolated with vessel tape. The median sacral artery must be ligated (Fig. 9).

The external iliac vessels should be dissected and freed from the tumor. When the external iliac vessels are sacrificed, the reconstruction should be performed first.

The internal iliac artery is usually located beneath the external iliac artery. The veins are located deeper than the arteries. Dissection can be attempted if the artery is located over the tumor. If dissection is impossible, the artery must be sacrificed.

Unilateral ligation of the internal iliac arteries does not cause ischemia of the pelvic organs. Branches running laterally (iliosacral, iliolumbar, superior and inferior gluteal, and obturator vessels) should usually be ligated. If dissection is possible, the superior gluteal artery can sometimes be preserved. All of the branches that run medially should also be ligated. It is frequently difficult to dissect the deeper branches of the internal iliac artery and vein, especially in the case of a large tumor. In such cases, the internal iliac artery and vein can be addressed through the posterior approach after the osteotomy is performed. The superior gluteal artery should be carefully dissected because it can easily be injured, and its hemostasis may be difficult. When the dissection is difficult, it should be managed through the posterior approach.

There is an extensive network of veins around the internal iliac vein, making it easily injured. If bleeding is uncontrollable, the surgery must be suspended, and a massive sponge should be packed into the wound. The surgical outcome will not be as good. To avoid such a complication, a wide exposure is recommended. If both distal and proximal portions of the injured vein can be compressed, the tear can be repaired.

When the dissection of the internal iliac artery is extended up to the greater sciatic notch, the anterior aspect of the sacroiliac joint can be exposed. Deeper vessels may be left undisturbed because they can be managed through the posterior approach. The psoas and iliacus muscles should be transected if necessary. If any nerve roots are affected, they should now be severed if possible. Usually, the L5 nerve root runs just on the sacroiliac joint (Fig. 10). The osteotomy line of the sacroiliac joint is marked by the placement of several Kirschner wires, as shown in Fig. 11. It is quite difficult to define the true osteotomy line through the posterior approach. The anterior approach is necessary to define the landmarks for the osteotomy. A Mickliz sponge or silicon plate should be left in place to protect the vessels on the anterior osteotomy line (Fig. 12).

The upper osteotomy line at L5/S1 or above is then dissected. The segmental spinal artery and vein are ligated and transected. The anterior aspect of the upper osteotomy level should be widely dissected. The nerve roots to be sacrificed are also cut. As much of the intervertebral disc as possible is excised at the intended

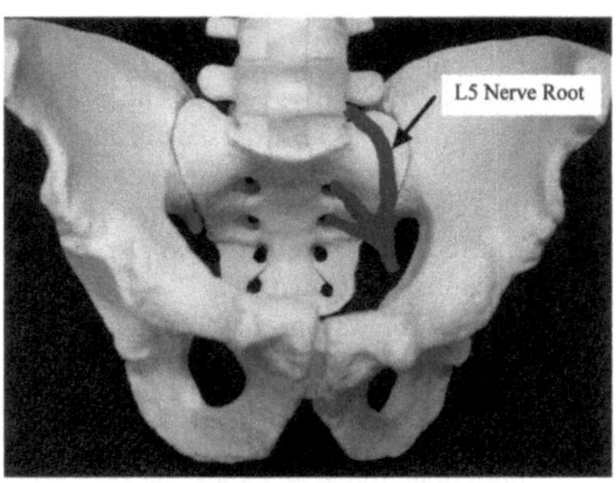

FIG. 10. Location of the spinal nerve roots. The L5 nerve root runs along the sacroiliac joint. This may be a good landmark

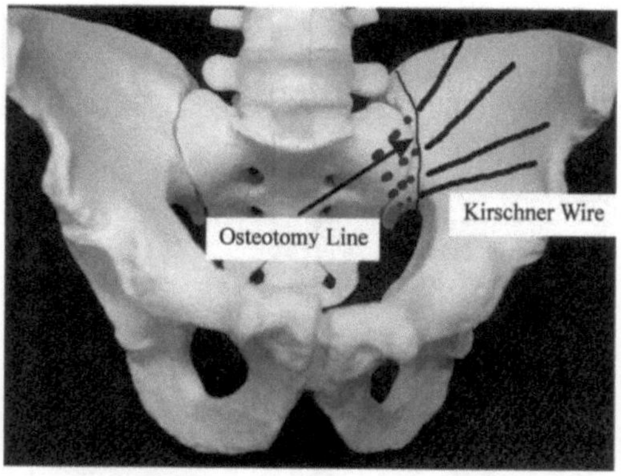

FIG. 11. Kirschner wires indicating the osteotomy line. Several Kirschner wires are introduced on the line of the osteotomy to guide the osteotome

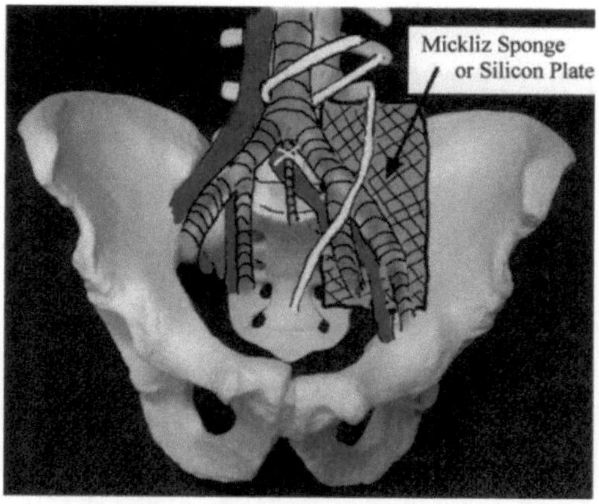

FIG. 12. Protection of the major vessels. A Mickliz sponge or a silicon plate is placed beneath the vessels to protect them from the osteotome, which is driven from the posterior approach

cut level (Fig. 13). The upper cut level is also covered with a sponge or a silicon plate.

The sacrum cannot be resected by the anterior approach only.

Total Sacrectomy

A combination of the anterior and posterior sacral approaches is essential for total sacrectomy. The position of the patient must be changed intraoperatively. The incision of the anterior approach is closed, and must be completely covered. The patient is then placed in the prone position, and scrubbing and draping are repeated in the usual manner. The posterior sacral approach is performed as described previously.

The lateral aspect of the sacrum and the greater sciatic notch should be widely exposed. The piriformis muscle is cut, piece-by-piece, through the posterior approach. The posterior aspect of the sacroiliac joint is widely exposed, and the locations of the landmark Kirschner wires must be confirmed. With a sponge or silicon plate serving as a guard in the anterior iliosacral region, as confirmed from the sciatic notch, the

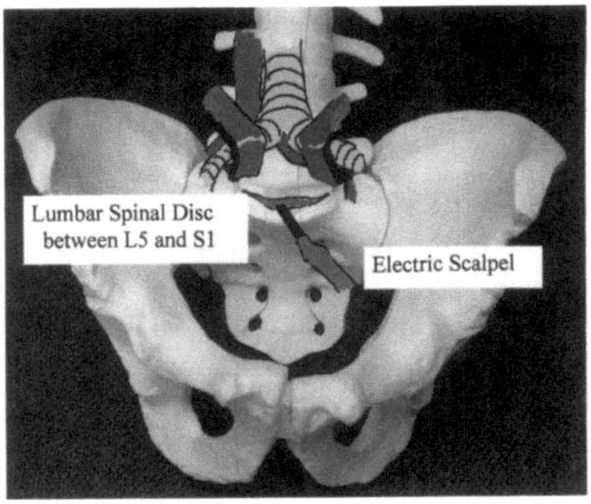

FIG. 13. Dissection of the upper resection level. As much of the intervertebral disc as possible is excised at the L5/S1 level

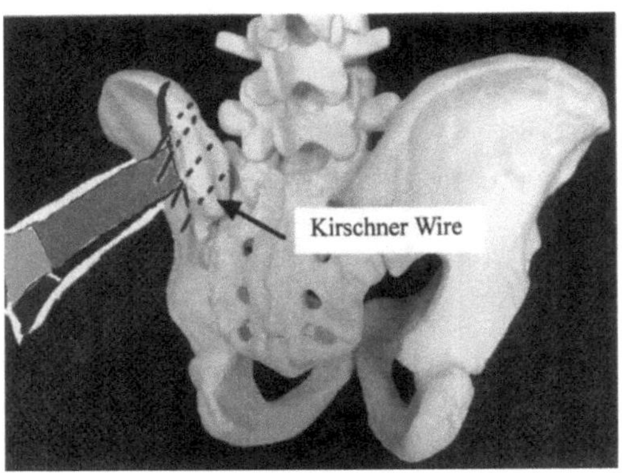

FIG. 14. Final osteotomy. Osteotomy of the lateral side of the sacrum or ilium is carried out with an osteotome along the Kirschner wires. The guiding Kirschner wires are used to ensure accuracy

lateral side of the sacrum or sacroiliac joint can be osteotomized safely. The insertion of the erector spinae muscle should be transected to expose the posterior aspect of the L5 vertebral body. The spine should be widely exposed up to the Mickliz sponge or silicon plate.

The laminectomy is carried out in the usual manner. The dural tube is ligated and cut cleanly at the intended amputation level. Osteotomy of both lateral sides of the sacrum or ilium is carried out with an osteotome along the Kirschner wires, or with a Gigli saw (Fig. 14).

Before completing the discotomy, a temporary internal fixation between the ilium and the spine must be applied otherwise separation of the spine and the pelvis will occur. After the internal fixation is completed, the final discotomy is performed. The sacrum is now freed from the spine and the ilium. The proximal stump is elevated posteriorly and reflected distally. Blunt dissection between the rectum and sacrum (tumor) is carried out distally. Deeper vessels from the branch of the internal iliac vessels can be managed by reflecting the sacrum. The total sacrectomy is then completed.

Ilium

Ilioinguinal Approach

The ilioinguinal approach is used for resection of the ilium, and also for resection of a retroperitoneal soft tissue tumor. This approach is also used in an internal hemipelvectomy and an ischiopubic resection.

Surgical Procedure

The usual preoperative preparation of the bowel should be carried out. The patient is placed in the lateral position with the affected side up. The entire affected limb should be scrubbed and draped in the usual manner. The genital and perineal areas must be carefully sterilized and draped. The skin incision is made along the inguinal band from the symphysis pubis to the anterior superior iliac spine (Fig. 15). The incision can then be extended posteriorly along the iliac wing (posterior iliac approach) or obliquely upward along the twelfth rib (oblique abdominal approach).

The abdominal muscles are transected with an electric knife in line with the skin incision (Fig. 16). The retroperitoneal space can usually be exposed without difficulty since fatty tissue exists in this space (Fig. 17). The superior epigastric artery, deep circumflex iliac artery, and superficial circumflex iliac artery should be ligated and severed (Fig. 18). In a male patient, the spermatic cord must be managed carefully. The inguinal canal is not usually opened. It is mobile on the pubic bone, and can be retracted medially. The location of the greater sciatic notch should be confirmed by palpation, or exposed if necessary.

When the tumor is exposed outside the iliacus muscle, a transperitoneal approach is necessary, and the peritoneum can be used as a barrier for the tumor. In such instances, however, replacement of the external iliac vessels will be necessary.

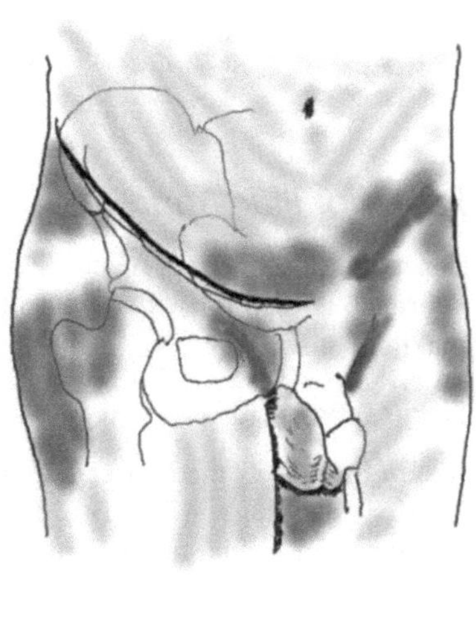

FIG. 15. Skin incision for the ilioinguinal approach. The incision is made along the inguinal band from the symphysis pubis to the anterior superior iliac spine

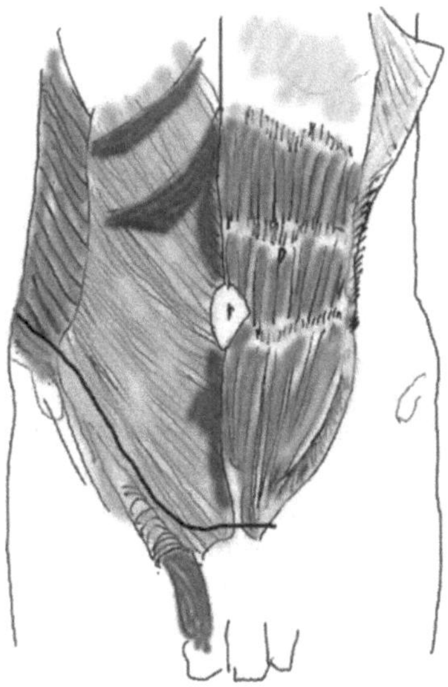

FIG. 16. Transection of the abdominal muscles. These are transected piece by piece with an electric knife

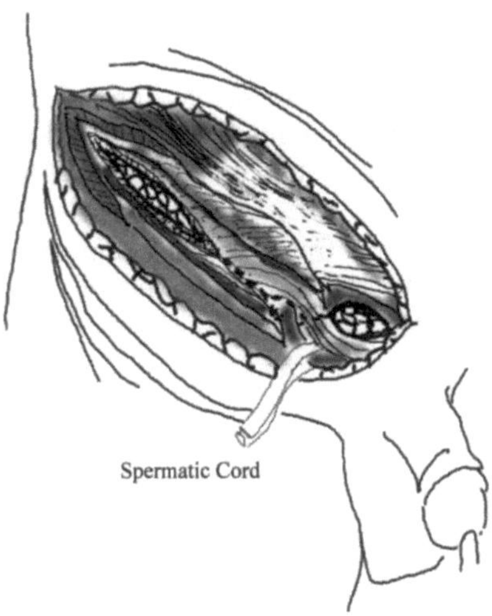

FIG. 17. Exposure of the retroperitoneal space. Fatty tissue is the landmark of the retroperitoneal space, which is easily exposed by blunt dissection. The spermatic cord is isolated with tape

Posterior Iliac Approach

The posterior iliac approach is a modification of the ilioinguinal approach. This approach is used for wider exposure of the posterior sacroiliac joint and the gluteus maximus muscle.

Surgical Procedure

A skin incision is made over the iliac wing, and is extended distally to the posterior inferior iliac spine (Fig. 19). The incision can be extended toward the greater trochanter or ischial tubercle in order to expose the hip joint.

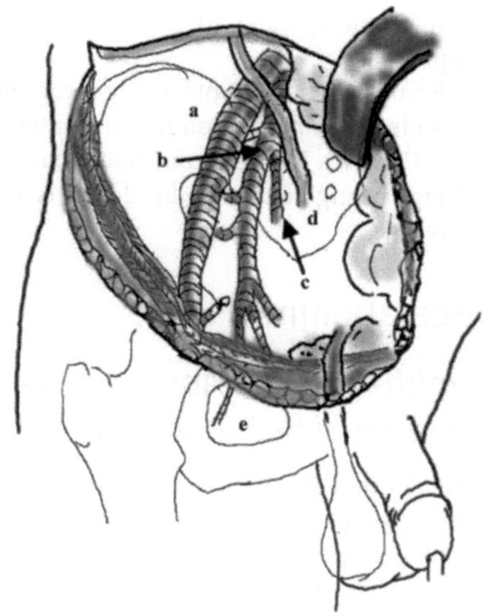

FIG. 18. Exposure of the major vessels. *a*, external iliac artery; *b*, internal iliac artery; *c*, lateral sacral artery; *d*, ureter; *e*, obturator artery. The intrapelvic branches of the external iliac artery can be ligated and severed

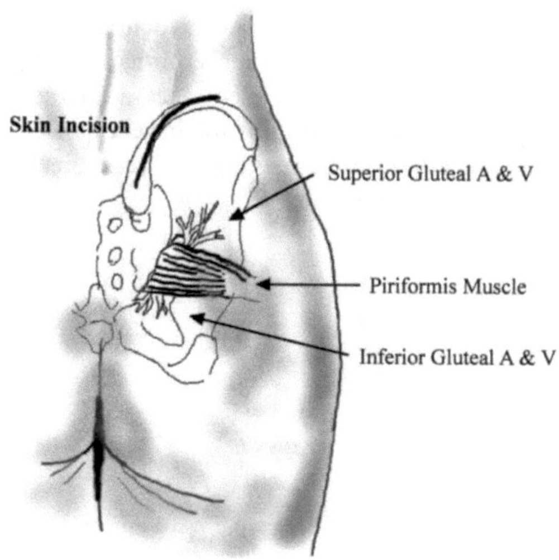

FIG. 19. Posterior iliac approach. The skin incision is made over the iliac wing, and is extended distally to the posterior inferior iliac spine

Resection of the Ilium

Resection of the ilium can be performed through the ilioinguinal and posterior iliac approaches. If the tumor has expanded outside the ilium, the gluteal muscles must be resected with the tumor. The distal portion of the muscles is cut at the margin of the wide excision. If this does not expose the tumor, the muscle can be detached from the iliac wing and reflected distally to a level sufficient to expose the tumor. The iliac bone is then widely exposed. The ilium can be osteotomized at any level through this approach.

Reconstruction is not usually recommended. However, we have experienced a case of wide bowel herniation into the anterior thigh after a simple resection of the ilium (see Chap. 7). We have concluded that the soft tissues of the inguinal region must be always be tightened. If the defect is too large, a marlex mesh sheet is useful for coverage.

Acetabulum

Smith–Peterson Approach and a Modification of Internal Hemipelvectomy

The Smith–Peterson anterior approach may be helpful in the case of a benign tumor, and when performing a curettage procedure. This approach is not described in this book because it has been covered in detail in many other texts.

In the event of a malignant bone tumor and wide resection, a modified approach for an internal hemipelvectomy (i.e., ilioinguinal, posterior iliac, or posterior ischial approaches) may be necessary. Care must be taken to preserve the blood supply to the skin flap. The two major suppliers of blood to the buttock skin are the lateral circumflex femoral artery and both the superior and inferior gluteal arteries. A tensor fascia lata or gluteus maximus myocutaneous flap is ideal. If a fasciocutaneous flap is needed, an L-shaped skin incision may result in necrosis of the edge of the flap (see Case 15 in Chap. 10). In such cases, a double-door skin incision may be safely used (Fig. 20), although we do not have experience of this incision. Campanacci and Capanna (1991) and Enneking and Dunham (1978) have reported a different approach for the acetabulum.

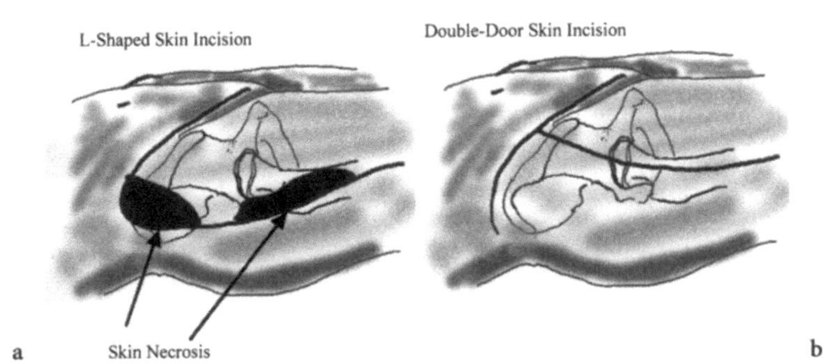

FIG. 20. Necrosis of a posterior gluteal fasciocutaneous flap. **a** An L-shaped skin incision resulted in necrosis of the edge of the flap. **b** A double-door skin incision may be safe in such cases, but we have no experience of this method

Pubis

Transperineal Approach and Ilioinguinal Approach

The transperineal and ilioinguinal approaches are used for resection of the upper rami, body, and lower rami of the pubis (Campanacci and Capanna 1991). The ischium cannot be exposed through this approach.

Surgical Procedure

The ilioinguinal approach has been described above. With the transperineal approach (Fig. 21), the patient is placed in the lithotomy position. Sterile scrubbing and draping are performed in the usual manner. In the female patient, the major labia are temporarily sutured together. The perineal area should be carefully sterilized. Both an ilioinguinal approach and a straight perineal approach can be used. The ilioinguinal approach can be elongated to the contralateral side to obtain wider exposure of the pubic symphysis and pubic angle (Fig. 22).

A perineal skin incision is made along the lower rami of the pubis. The incision can be extended to the medial thigh to expose the adductor muscle.

The inner side of the pubis and symphysis is first dissected. The urinary bladder can usually be freed by blunt digital dissection (Fig. 23). The pubic angle is easily exposed, and an elevator can be introduced without initiating bleeding. The obturator artery and nerve are also identified. The artery is ligated and severed. The nerve

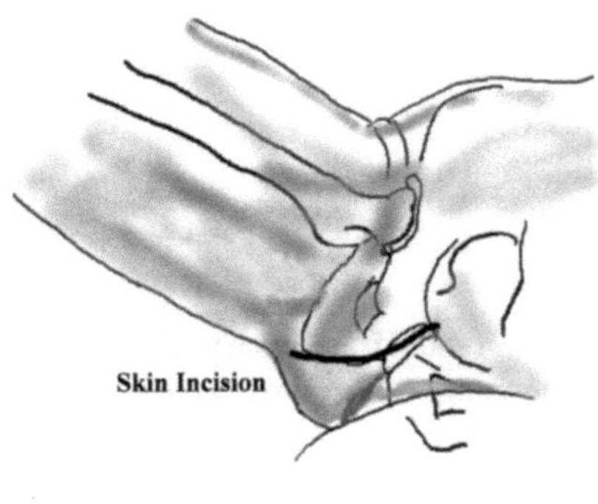

FIG. 21. Skin incision for the transperineal approach. The incision is made along the lower rami of the pubis

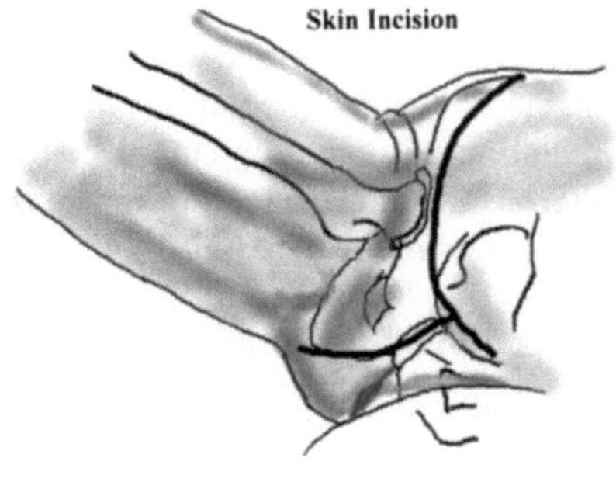

FIG. 22. A combination of the ilioinguinal and transperineal approaches

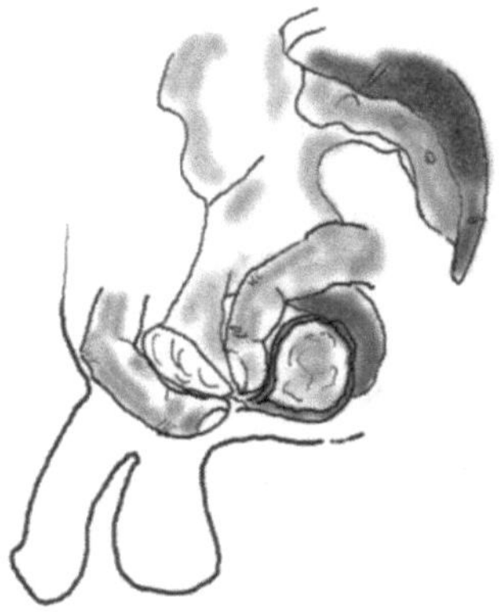

FIG. 23. Dissection of the urinary bladder. The urinary bladder can usually be freed by blunt finger dissection

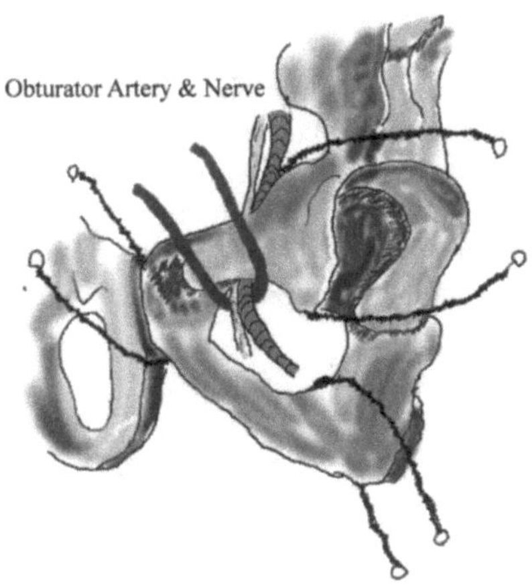

FIG. 24. Triple osteotomy of the pubis. The obturator muscle, pectineus muscle, adductors, and gracilis muscle are severed. Dissection of the urogenital diaphragm and the muscles of the floor of the pelvis should be done after triple osteotomy

is transected if necessary. The nerve should be reconstructed with a sural nerve graft. The prognosis for its recovery is good. The location of the obturator foramen is confirmed.

The adductor, pectineus, and internal and external obturator muscles are transected at the level of the wide excision. A triple osteotomy of the symphysis, upper rami, and lower rami is performed with a Gigli saw (Fig. 24). The symphysis can also be cut with an electric knife. The pubis is then connected by the urogenital membrane only. The membrane is carefully cut, piece-by-piece, by retracting the osteotomized bone. If there is insufficient margin in the membrane, resection of the urethra and urinary diversion will be necessary.

Resection of the Pubis

The entire pubis can be resected using this approach. There are only a few reports in the literature describing reconstruction of the pubis. Most authors insist that bony reconstruction is not necessary. However, some patients without pubic reconstruction complain of pain in the ipsilateral sacroiliac joint. Therefore, reconstruction of the pubis is usually unnecessary, but if there is the risk of an unstable pelvic ring, reconstruction of the pubis should be performed using a free fibula graft. The stump of the urogenital membrane can be left free. Generally, no vesicorectal problems occur.

Ischium

Posterior Ischial Approach

This approach can be used only for curettage or subperiosteal resection of the ischium. When a wider resection of the ischium is necessary, the combination of an ilioinguinal approach and a transperineal approach must be used. A lateral position is recommended, as in the case of a hemipelvectomy.

Surgical Procedure

The patient is placed in the decubitus position. Scrubbing and draping are performed in the usual manner. A slightly wavy skin incision is made over the ischium from the posterior inferior iliac spine to the ischial tubercle (Fig. 25). The wound is deepened and the lower third of the gluteus maximus is severed. If wider exposure is necessary, the sciatic nerve should be identified and retracted safely. The external obturator and gemellus muscles are transected on the ischium. This will provide exposure of the entire posterior aspect of the ischium.

Resection of the Ischium

The usual preoperative bowel preparation must be performed. The patient is placed in the lateral position, and the entire affected limb is scrubbed and draped in the usual

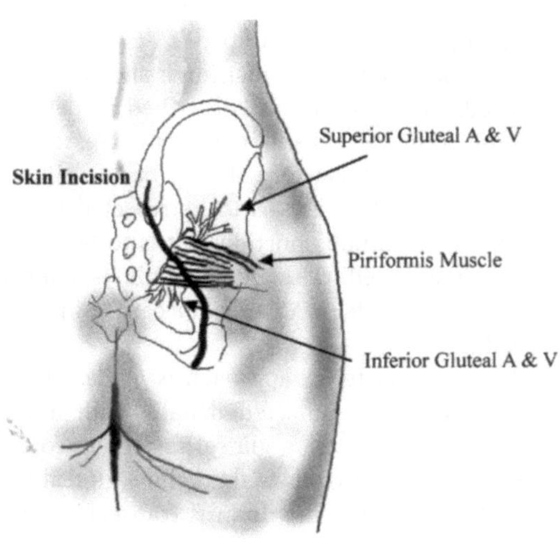

FIG. 25. Skin incision for the posterior ischial approach. A slightly wavy skin incision is made over the ischium from the posterior inferior iliac spine to the ischial tubercle

manner. The perineal area should be carefully sterilized and draped. A combination of the posterior ischial approach, ilioinguinal approach, and transperineal approach is used. When it is possible to preserve the lower rami of the pubis, the transperineal approach is unnecessary. The gemellus and internal obturator muscles should be transected inside the pelvis through the ilioinguinal approach. Then these muscles are again severed distally through the posterior approach. The obturator artery and nerve are also cut if necessary. The posterior approach is then performed. The piriformis muscle and other short rotators are transected at their insertions. The sacrotuberous ligament is severed carefully. The entire ischium can then be resected.

Hemipelvectomy

A conventional hemipelvectomy is not considered in this book because the procedure is described in detail in many texts. The particular procedure of an internal hemipelvectomy is explained here. This is a special modification of hemipelvectomy for limb salvage.

Internal Hemipelvectomy

The ipsilateral limb may be preserved in many patients with a tumor involving the hemipelvis. In general, the affected limb can be saved if the external iliac artery is preserved and a good skin flap is obtained. This approach is a combination of the ilioinguinal, posterior iliac, and ischial approaches. Special attention must be paid to the management of the femoral and sciatic nerves. The femoral nerve, in particular, is very tight and is damaged more easily than the sciatic nerve.

Surgical Procedure

The usual preoperative preparation of the bowel should be carried out. The patient is placed in the lateral position with the affected side up. The entire affected limb should be scrubbed and draped in the usual manner. The genital and perineal areas must be carefully sterilized and draped.

The shape of the skin incision is shown in Fig. 26. At first, the ilioinguinal approach is used. The procedure is described in detail. The purpose of this procedure is to expose both external and internal iliac vessels. The femoral nerve, the obturator nerve, and the obturator artery should be identified. The obturator artery and nerve are transected if the pubis is to be resected together. The iliacus muscle is transected in its myotendinous portion if it is to be resected. The greater sciatic notch should also be exposed. The pubic angle is exposed after blunt digital dissection of the urinary bladder. An elevator can be introduced into the angle without initiating bleeding.

Next, the posterior approach is made. The gluteus maximus is detached from its iliac origin, and reflected distally with a musculocutaneous flap. If the gluteus maximus is resected, a gluteal fasiocutaneous flap may be risky. However, we have no experience of cases with a whole gluteal fasciocutaneous flap. The paravertebral muscle attached to the ilium is transected. The gluteus medius is detached from its origin if possible. If the tumor has invaded the muscle, it must be severed at the

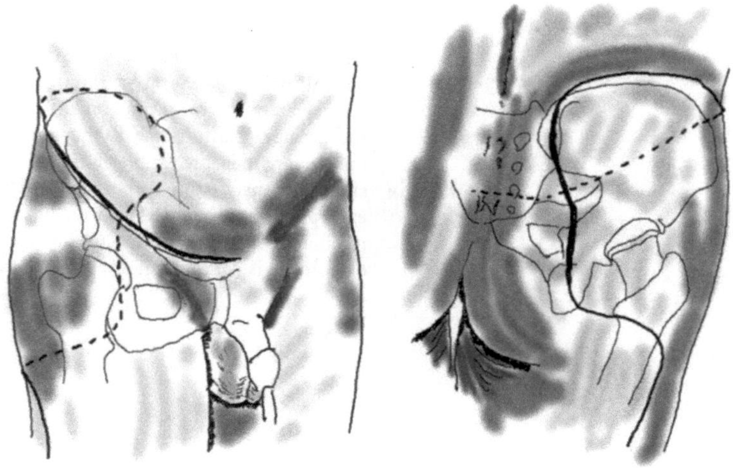

FIG. 26. Skin incision for an internal hemipelvectomy. This skin incision is a combination of the ilioinguinal, posterior iliac, and posterior ischial approaches. The final line is extended to the greater trochanter, and goes down along the femur

femoral insertion and sacrificed. The gluteus minimus may be managed, as well as the gluteus medius. The tensor fascia lata muscle can be severed at any level. Usually, the greater sciatic notch is easily exposed. The sciatic nerve, superior and inferior gluteal arteries, and piriformis muscle are exposed. They can be preserved if the tumor is not exposed outside the cortex of the notch. If the tumor is exposed, the piriformis muscle, superior gluteal artery, and inferior gluteal artery must be resected as a barrier. We have no clear evidence of the true blood supply to the gluteus maximus, but even when both gluteal arteries were ligated, the gluteus maximus musculocutaneous flap survived in the few cases we have met. Then the sacrospinous ligament and the sacrotuberous ligament are transected as shown in the section on sacral amputation (see Fig. 2).

Hip disarticulation is then carried out. The short rotators are cut at any level. The tendon of the iliopsoas can be severed if necessary. The adductors, gracilis, pectineus, hamstrings, and rectus femoris muscles are severed at any level. The joint capsule of the hip joint is cut, and the joint is dislocated. If the joint is contaminated by the tumor, the neck of the femur is osteotomized to resect the joint together.

Now the hemipelvis is connected by the symphysis, urogenital membrane, and sacroiliac joint, only. The symphysis pubis is cut with an electric scalpel or a wire saw. Then the sacroiliac joint is osteotomized with a wire saw, as illustrated (Fig. 27). The hemipelvis can now be moved. The branches of the internal iliac artery and vein are easily managed (Fig. 28), and the urogenital membrane and the muscles of the pelvic floor are easily transected. Finally, the internal hemipelvectomy is completed.

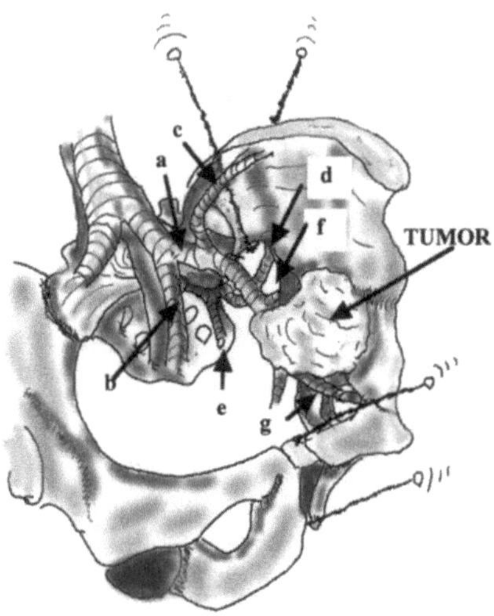

FIG. 27. Anatomy of the major vessels and osteotomy. *a*, internal iliac artery; *b*, external iliac artery; *c*, iliolumbar artery; *d*, superior gluteal artery; *e*, lateral sacral artery; *f*, inferior gluteal artery; *g*, obturator artery. Clearance of the greater sciatic notch is the most important maneuver. It is preferable if this is carried out simultaneously from both an intrapelvic and an extrapelvic approach. Deep branches of the internal iliac vessels may be left unmanaged until the osteotomy is carried out

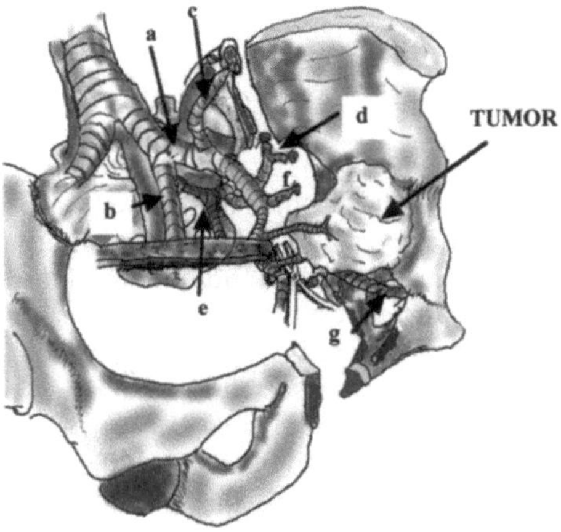

FIG. 28. Management of deep-seated vessels. *a*, internal iliac artery; *b*, external iliac artery; *c*, iliolumbar artery; *d*, superior gluteal artery; *e*, lateral sacral artery; *f*, inferior gluteal artery; *g*, obturator artery. Deep-seated vessels are relatively easy to manage after osteotomy

Retroperitoneal Tumor

Extraperitoneal Approach

Two major extraperitoneal approaches are used. One method involves a combination of an ilioinguinal approach and an oblique abdominal approach, as mentioned in the description of approaches to the ilium. The other method involves a pararectal approach (Fig. 29), which is usually used for inguinal lymph node dissection. This approach can only provide limited exposure, and is not indicated for the removal of a large tumor.

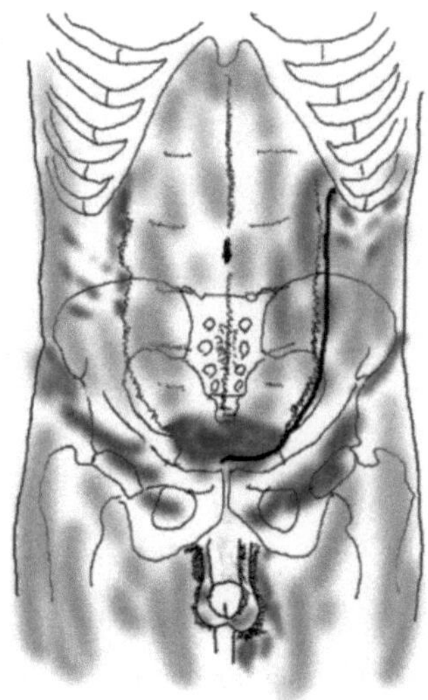

Fig. 29. Skin incision for the pararectal approach. The incision is made along the margin of the rectus abdominis muscle

Lateral Extraperitoneal Approach (Combination of the Ilioinguinal and Oblique Abdominal Approaches)

Exposure to the level of the body of L3 can be obtained with the lateral extraperitoneal approach. Exposure extending to higher levels can be made by resection of the lower rib and incision of the diaphragm.

The involvement of the ureter, urinary bladder, and external iliac vessels must be checked preoperatively, and a urologist and a cardiovascular surgeon should always be consulted. An ipsilateral nephrectomy may be necessary in some cases. If involvement of the external iliac vessels is suspected, preparations for vascular reconstruction should be made.

In many instances, reconstruction of the external iliac artery and vein is necessary. In such cases, the ilioinguinal approach should be extended downward to the anterior thigh. A T-shaped skin incision could also be made (Fig. 30). The external iliac artery can be replaced by an artificial vessel. However, the use of an artificial vein is less satisfactory. Venous drainage into the contralateral external iliac vein is effectively obtained by a graft of its major saphenous vein. This procedure is presented in detail in the section on the reconstruction of venous drainage after sacrificing the external iliac vein, in Chap. 7, and in Case 13 in Chap. 10.

Surgical Procedure

The patient is placed in the lateral position with the affected side up. An ilioinguinal approach is made first, and the skin incision is elongated between the iliac wing and the 12th rib. The retroperitoneal space is exposed by the ilioinguinal approach, and the abdominal muscles are cut in line with an oblique abdominal skin incision. The dissection of the pelvic cavity and the anterior aspect of the spine are described in the sections on the anterior sacral approach and total sacrectomy in this chapter. Wide exposure of the major vessels up to the lower abdominal aorta is also possible.

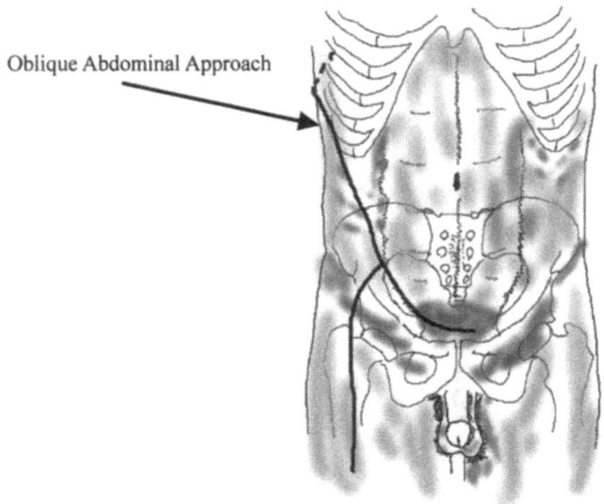

FIG. 30. Oblique abdominal approach and T-shaped approach. The skin incision is made at the 12th rib, and goes down toward the anterior superior iliac spine. It connects with the skin incision of the ilioinguinal approach. An anterior thigh skin incision is added to make a T-shape

If vascular reconstruction is necessary and more surgical time is required, vascular reconstruction of the external iliac artery and vein should be performed first. The internal iliac vessels can be ligated and transected if necessary.

Transperitoneal Approach (Abdominoinguinal Approach)

A colostomy is sometimes necessary. If so, the abdominoinguinal approach is recommended (Karakousis 1982, 1984). This approach can provide wide exposure of the pelvic cavity. An abdominal midline skin incision is used for the laparotomy. This incision can be extended downward, across the inguinal band, and into the anterior thigh. The femoral vessels and nerve are then exposed. After the rectus muscle is transected and the lateral one-third of the inguinal ligament is detached from the iliac fascia, it is possible to obtain complete exposure of the ipsilateral side of the pelvis. If the tumor adheres to the posterior peritoneum, the major vessels and ureter can be exposed by severing the posterior peritoneum.

References

Campanacci M, Capanna R (1991) Pelvic resections: the Rizzoli Institute experience. Orthop Clin North Am 22:65–86

Enneking WF, Dunham WK (1978) Resection and reconstruction for primary neoplasms involving the innominate bone. J Bone Joint Surg Am 60:731–746

Karakousis CP (1982) Exposure and reconstruction in the lower portions of the retroperitoneum and abdominal wall. Arch Surg 117:840–844

Karakousis CP (1984) The abdominoinguinal incision in limb salvage and resection of pelvic tumors. Cancer 54:2543–2548

Ozaki T, Hillmann A, Winkelmann W (1997) Surgical treatment of sacrococcygeal chordoma. J Sur Oncol 64:274–279

Samson IR, Springfield DS, Suit HD, Mankin HJ (1993) Operative treatment of sacrococcygeal chordoma. A review of twenty-one cases. J Bone Joint Surg Am 75:1476–1484

Stener B, Gunterberg B (1978) High amputation of the sacrum for extirpation of tumors. Principles and technique. Spine 3:351–366

Waisman M, Kligman M, Roffman M (1997) Posterior approach for radical excision of sacral chordoma. Int Orthop 21:181–184

Chapter 6
Reconstruction

Reconstructive Surgery After Wide Resection of Pelvic Tumors

HIDEAKI E. TAKAHASHI

Summary. Reconstruction of the pelvic ring after the removal of a bone tumor is necessary to transmit the weight of the trunk to the lower extremities. This is important in order for the patient to be able to sit, stand, and walk, with or without an external support such as a cane or a pair of crutches. Our initial experiences with reconstruction are described in this chapter. Bone grafts, with or without internal hardware, are needed for the reconstruction of a bone defect after the removal of a tumor involving the unilateral or bilateral sacroiliac joints, and for any defect of the ilium between the sacroiliac joint and the hip joint. A bone graft may not be needed for a continuation of the osseous ring with a defect at the symphysis pubis when the bilateral sacroiliac joints are mechanically intact. Various procedures for the reconstruction of a defect after resection surgery are discussed.

Key words. Bone defect, Pelvic ring, Sacroiliac joint, Symphysis pubis, Strut

General Principles

Procedures for the resection of a primary bone tumor involving the innominate bone and/or the sacrum can be divided into marginal excision, wide excision, radical resection, and hemipelvectomy (Enneking and Dunham 1978; Enneking 1983). Later Enneking and Dunham proposed the concept of grading benign and malignant musculoskeletal tumors in order to help in decisions about suitable treatments, and to make meaningful comparisons of methods of treatment (Heare et al. 1989; Carnesale 1998). Enneking's grading system for benign and malignant musculoskeletal tumors consists of the grade (G), the site (T), and the metastasis (M). Benign tumors are classified as stage 1, 2, or 3, and malignant tumors are stage I, II, or III. These stages are subdivided into A or B according to grade, site, and metastasis (Heare et al. 1989). With the improved anatomic staging classification now available, and the effectiveness of adjuvant therapies, emphasis has been placed on surgical resections aimed at salvaging limbs. A precise radiographic, anatomical localization of the tumor is required before planning both the surgery and the biopsy, in order to achieve a definitive diagnosis and an adequate margin. Even though magnetic resonance imaging is very helpful in showing the extent of a bone tumor preoperatively, the margin should be determined by a careful analysis of the specimen postoperatively. The following terms were used by Enneking and Dunham. *Intralesional margins* result when the dissection passes through the lesion. *Marginal margins* result when the dissection passes within reactive tissue contiguous with the lesion. *Wide margins* result when the dissection is carried out entirely through normal tissue at a distance from the lesion. *Radical margins* result when all normal tissues of all the compartments involved are removed from their origin to the insertion. Procedures to remove a tumor with no amputation are called *local excisions* or *resections*. These are limb-sparing procedures. Using these definitions, local resections may be designated *marginal*, *wide*, or *radical* depending on the margins achieved. If intralesional margins result, the procedure is called *debulking*.

Bone and soft tissue tumors of the innominate bone and the sacrum are included in this series. Pelvic resections were classified as being in one of three major anatomical regions using a modified Enneking classification of the innominate bone (Enneking and Dunham 1978; Enneking 1983; Campanacci et al. 1987; Campanacci 1990): (I) iliac, (II) periacetabular, (III) ischiopubic, and the sacrum (Stener and Gunterberg 1978). A capital "A" indicates a more aggressive resection: (IA) the buttock is resected en bloc with the iliac wing; (IIA) the proximal femur and hip capsule are resected with the periacetabulum; (IIIA) the femoral neurovascular bundle is resected with the pubic rami. Some large lesions occupy more than one region of the innominate bone and sacrum. Each region of the innominate bone is subdivided into four categories according to the extension of the resection (Campanacci and Capanna 1991; Campanacci 1999).

When treating a tumor of the pelvis, surgical resection, radiation therapy, and adjuvant chemotherapy should all be considered according to the tumor's pathology, whether it is benign or malignant, its sensitivity to radiation or drug therapy, and its three-dimensional anatomical progression. Curettage, resection, or irradiation alone must then be selected (Sanjay et al. 1993). Although preradiation and postradiation therapy is required for the control of some tumors, or in some cases to maintain a higher level of quality of life, surgical resection may often be the first treatment choice. Any operative treatment in the pelvic region will create a defect, and this will result in a need for reconstruction of the continuity and stability of the trunk to the pelvis, and of the pelvic ring and pelvis to the lower extremities. This would make it possible for the patient to sit, stand, and walk, thereby maintaining the essential activities of daily living.

The method of reconstruction after resection of the tumor varies according to the anatomical location of the lesion and the extent of the defect. Enneking's classification of resection (Enneking and Dunham 1978) is still useful in planning the appropriate reconstruction to correspond to the type of resection performed. Since this report, various endoprostheses for hip joints, hardware for internal fixation, and spinal instruments have become available, as well as external fixaters (Campanacci and Capanna 1991; O'Connor and Sim 1992; Osaka 1995).

The method of reconstruction has to be customized to each patient according to the location and nature of the defect. The quality of the patient's life must be considered, and the resection of part of the pelvic bone tumor may have to be marginal. Reconstruction involves not only osseous tissue, but also soft tissue, including skin and muscle, as well as intrapelvic organs such as the urogenital organs. When an orthopedic surgeon decides on the extent of a resection of a pelvic tumor and surrounding tissue, they should estimate the size of the defect preoperatively. Previous case reports describing the reconstructive procedures and their outcome may be very helpful in planning a new case.

In each section of this chapter, our experience with reconstructions of the pelvic ring will be described first, and then a discussion of the reconstructive procedures will follow. Skin coverage using microsurgical techniques with various skin grafts and flaps will be discussed in the next chapter.

Reconstruction After Resection of the Iliac Region

Wedge resection of the ilium (a type-I resection), including a bone tumor, does not interrupt the pelvic ring, and therefore does not usually require reconstruction using a bone graft. However, when all of the ilium is resected, with subsequent interruption of the pelvic ring, or after a type-IA resection, the defect may require reconstruction.

Planning

A bone defect created by the resection of a tumor in the ilium or sacrum, including the sacroiliac joint, necessitates reconstruction of the continuity of the pelvic ring. Without this continuity, the patient is unable to support their body weight, and may experience pain when walking. The sacroiliac joint should be able to withstand both the compressive loads encountered in the stance phase of the gait cycle, as well as the tensile loads in the swing phase. In order to regain bony continuity, fibular grafting with autogenous bone, supplemented with a Harrington compression rod (used for scoliosis surgery), was selected to resist the compressive loads, and a threaded sacral bar fixed with a hook and nut was chosen to resist the tension loads. The size and geometry of the bone graft were determined by the biomechanical demands of the patient.

Procedure

After tumor resection, when the size of the defect has been determined, autogenous fibula bone grafts are harvested with as much length as possible. These are suitable for transmitting the mechanical loads from the trunk to the lower extremities. In our series, a distraction rod from the Harrington system was placed obliquely. Then two or three segments of fibula, fashioned to almost the same length as the defect, were placed diagonally between the L3, L4, and L5 vertebral bodies, the transverse processes, and the ilium (as demonstrated in case 1), or between the sacrum and the ilium (as shown in case 3). A 5-mm-deep cross-slit was made at each end of each fibula graft segment before it was inserted in the cancellous bone of the vertebral body in order to increase the surface area of the cortical bone for easier revascularization. The fibula was placed into the cancellous portion of the sacrum and ilium, parallel to the distraction rod. The compression rod with a hook at each end was also placed into both the sacrum and the ilium. A compressive force was then applied to the segments of the fibula and to the distraction rod. In addition, segments of iliac bone harvested from the contralateral ilium were put in place and fixed with stainless steel wire.

Outcome

In case 3, the patient began to walk with partial weight-bearing within 6 weeks after resection surgery, and with full weight-bearing at the end of 3 months. The fibular grafts and segments of ilium were gradually homogenized and fused with the sacrum and ilium.

Discussion

Resection of the ilium, the sacroiliac joint, and the sacral wing resulted in the interruption of the pelvic ring. The use of free autogenous fibular grafts, together with Harrington rods in both distraction and compression, were sufficient for gait without external support in this series (case 3). The grafted fibula was 12 cm long. Campanacci et al. (1987) reported that after complete resection of the ilium in children, progressive deformity with shortening will occur, and the defect should be reconstructed with a bone graft. In addition, the acetabulum and remaining ilium hinges on the symphysis pubis, and it gradually and spontaneously approaches the sacrum, resulting in a relatively painless condition. Vascularised fibular grafting between the sacrum and ilium, just above the acetabulum, has been advocated (Leung 1992; Yajima et al. 1992).

Reconstruction After Periacetabular Resection

When the tumor involves the acetabular region, a number of reconstructive methods are available. When only a portion of the acetabulum is resected, the defect may be reconstructed with autogenous bone grafts. When the lesion involves the entire acetabulum, a total acetabular resection is needed (type II), and the proximal femur and hip capsule, together with the periacetabulum, are resected (type IIA). It is then necessary to choose between arthrodesis, arthoplasty, and resection arthroplasty.

Planning

Periacetabular resection may be divided into intraarticular or extraarticular removal. The former involves resection of the acetabulum with dislocation of the femoral head, while the latter includes resection of the proximal femur, which is removed en bloc with the acetabulum without opening the joint capsule. The extent and nature of a lesion in the acetabulum should be evaluated by computed tomography and magnetic resonance imaging, and diagnosed by biopsy as being either benign, aggressive, recurring benign, or malignant. The indication for the procedure can then be made. It should be possible to obtain an adequate margin without sacrificing major neurovascular bundles, particularly the sciatic nerve. In malignant tumors, an adequate margin for resection is usually the same as that for a hindquarter amputation.

Procedure

In periacetabular resection, various methods should be considered, taking into account the diagnosis of the tumor, whether it is benign or malignant, the patient's age and occupation, and also the patient's need for flexion, stability, and durability. The possible surgical approaches were described in Chap. 5. When intraarticular resection is performed, the joint capsule is incised circularly and the femoral head is dislocated. When extraarticular resection is performed, the femoral neck is transected at its base, or the femoral shaft is osteotomized distal to the trochanters, without opening the joint. Endoprosthetic arthroplasty is performed for those needing flexion. If an arthrodesis is indicated, various methods should be considered such as an iliofemoral arthrodesis fixed internally with a screwed plate, an ischiofemoral arthrodesis, or an iliofemoral pseudoarthorosis, i.e., resection arthroplasty.

Outcome

An arthrodesis is indicated for patients who are working and require stability and durability. Endoprosthetic replacement of the hip joint is most suitable for those who sit most of the day and need flexion of the hip.

Discussion

In periacetabular excision of an Enneking's type II low grade intraosseous tumor involving the entire acetabulum and adjacent neck of the ilium, the ischium, and the lateral portion of the pubic rami, it is recommended that the femoral head be dislocated and preserved (Enneking and Dunham 1978). Wide resection of the hip joint en bloc, including the periacetabular bone, the acetabulum, the capsule, and the proximal femur, is needed when the tumor has invaded the hip joint.

Endoprosthetic replacements have been used for the reconstruction of a defect after tumor resection. Harrington (1981) reported the use of hip replacement arthroplasty in the case of a metastatic malignant tumor. A saddle prosthesis was implanted after the resection of a metastatic cystosarcoma and chondrosarcoma (van der Lei et al. 1992). A constrained hip prosthesis has been designed, and was used after resections of a chondrosarcoma, osteosarcoma, malignant fibrous histiocytoma, and metastatic bone tumor (Uchida et al. 1996). A nonconstrained custom-made pelvic prosthesis and a conventional Stanmore femoral prosthesis have been used for the reconstruction of a defect (Abudu et al. 1997). Campanacci and Capanna (1991) reported a reconstruction of the acetabulum with a shaped autograft, and of the femur with a modular endoprosthesis.

Arthrodesis between the ilium and the femoral head, or between the ischium and the femoral head, using an autogenous bone graft (Enneking and Dunham 1978; Osaka and Toriyama 1987; Campanacci et al. 1987; Campanacci and Capanna 1991; O'Connor and Sim 1989; Campanacci 1999), was found to be an excellent procedure for reconstruction because it was painless, durable, and stable (Enneking and Menendez 1987; Enneking et al. 1993). However, this procedure might result in a shortening of the limb, and require too much time to attain a rigid bony union. The recent development of improved instrumentation allows a more rigid fixation between the lower lumbar spine and the sacrum, through the innominate bone, to the proximal femur. This has shortened the time required for a bony union without the immobilization provided by casting. Furthermore, the reduction in limb length might be counterbalanced by increasing the femoral length by an external fixator (Ilizarov 1992; Kusuzaki et al. 1998).

Resection arthroplasty has been reported to be an alternative to drastic resection surgery (Steel 1978). The patients were immobilized with a double hip spica cast for 6 weeks. Most of the patients could walk without support, although they experienced a shortening of the limb, and exhibited telescoping of the femur and a Trendelenburg gait (Nilsonne et al. 1982). Kusuzaki et al. (1998) reported five cases, each treated with resection arthroplasty and maintained with an external fixator for 6 weeks after surgery. Leg-lengthening was performed simultaneously, since limb-shortening after resection was expected. Resection arthroplasty may prove to be a good alternative, although their series was too small, and the follow-up period was too short for a firm evaluation.

Allografts are available at a limited number of institutions, but we have not used them. Allografts (Langlais and Vielpeau 1989; Guest et al. 1990; Mnaymneth et al. 1997) and autoclaved (Harrington et al. 1986) or irradiated autografts of the pelvis have been used for hip reconstruction, but they require a long period of fixation until graft incorporation and full weight-bearing are achieved. Rosenberg and Mankin (1986) have described reconstructions using a pelvic osteochondral allograft with or without a hip prosthesis. The procedure may give an excellent functional result by restoring hip motion and preserving limb length, although it has been complicated by high rates of infection. These procedures were followed by total hip replacement, because rapid degeneration of the articular cartilage of the grafted acetabulum occurred.

The placement of a vascularized autograft of the ankle joint of an amputated limb might be another choice for reconstruction of the periacetabular resection, as described in Chap. 6, by H. Saito, this volume. However, the follow-up times were too short to evaluate the outcome of this procedure.

Reconstruction After Resection of the Ischiopubic Region

After the resection of a lesion in the anterior portion of the pelvis (type III), a reconstruction to transmit body weight is not usually necessary.

Planning

A bone defect resulting from the resection of a tumor in the region of the symphysis pubis necessitates reconstruction to prevent visceral herniation and to protect the intrapelvic organs, including the urinary bladder, urethra, and other abdominal viscera. When the sacroiliac joint is intact, the patient should have no difficulty with the weight-bearing ability of the hip joint without bony continuity of the pelvic ring at the symphysis pubis. Only skin coverage with subcutaneous supplementary fascia or a mesh-graft is needed to repair the defect.

Procedure

In our series, the tensor fascia latae was harvested from the lateral aspect of the thigh. The fascia was put in place and sutured to the surrounding tissue at the defect. A surgical mesh may be used instead of autogenous tissue. The skin may be covered using a local flap such as a groin flap, or a free vascularized flap, as described later in this chapter.

Outcome

In this series, a patient with a bone defect at the symphysis pubis, which was covered by a local groin flap, had no problem with herniation of the abdominal viscera (case 4). However, the patient needed to wear a tight girdle.

Discussion

No significant bony reconstruction is required after ischiopubic resection or bilateral pubic ramus excision (Enneking and Dunham 1978). When the external genitalia, together with the skin and subcutaneous tissue, can be preserved by reflecting them bilaterally from the symphysis and inferior pubic rami, soft tissue reconstruction is rarely needed. When only a portion of the bladder wall is excised, a simple plastic closure over the temporary catheter drainage is usually sufficient. When the tumor and its reactive zone involve the urethra and/or bladder, these have to be excised to obtain a wide margin. A multistage urogenital reconstruction is then required. When a total cystectomy is needed, the ureters are diverted transcutaneously or into a prepared loop of bowel. In our series (case 4), an ileal conduit was formed, and its function has been satisfactory for 17 years since the surgery.

Reconstruction After Resection of the Sacrum

Planning

A defect resulting from a total sacrectomy, or from the replacement of the sacrum by a tumor, would create bilateral instability of the sacroiliac joints. Patients complain of a sensation of the trunk sinking into the pelvis, as well as an inability to stand or walk. This necessitates a reconstruction of bilateral continuity and stability between the lumbar spine and the ilium. In order to connect the upper trunk and the pelvis, four supporting struts have been designed, with the fore strut positioned anterior to, and the hind strut positioned posterior to, the center axis of the lumbar spine on each side, as described in case 2.

Procedure

In our series, the hind struts were placed through a posterior midline approach using dual Harrington distraction rods. The upper hooks were inserted bilaterally into the L3 laminae, and the lower ends of the dual rods were supported with the eyelets and a sacral bar fixed between the bilateral ilia. The fore strut of the autogenous fibular graft was installed through an anterior retroperitoneal approach. To insert the fibula into the anteroinferior corner of the L3 vertebral body, a portion of the intervertebral disk between L3 and L4 was removed, and a groove for the fibula was made at the anterior side wall of the L4 vertebral body. The genitofemoral nerve was preserved, the psoas major muscle was retracted medially, the femoral nerve was retracted laterally, and a portion of the iliacus muscle was transected, exposing the pelvic rim of the ilium. The segment of fibula was fixed with two screws, with the upper screw placed into the L4 vertebral body and the lower one inserted into the pelvis. Another short segment of the fibula was grafted between the transverse process of L4 and the posterior iliac crest, requiring the partial removal of the insertion of the quadratus lumborum and iliacus muscles, and the iliolumbar ligament. The left fibular graft was placed between the L3 vertebral body and the left pelvic rim.

Outcome

In our series, after reestablishing the connection between the trunk and the pelvis with the four strut grafts (case 2), the subjective sensation of the trunk sinking into the pelvis ceased. This was also apparent radiographically. After the first series of operations, the patient could walk without the use of an external support, since the weight of his upper body was supported by the four strut grafts. Approximately a year and a half later, the remnant of the sacrum was resected owing to the recurrence of the tumor. The patient died from extensive bleeding from the iliac artery, which resulted from infection and a fragile artery after radiation therapy.

Discussion

The strength of the pelvis after major amputation of the sacrum was determined in an experimental study of 15 cadaveric pelves by Gunterberg et al. (1976). The pelvic ring was weakened by approximately 30% after resection of the sacrum between S1 and S2, and by 50% after resection 1 cm below the sacral promontory. Gunterberg et al. concluded that it would be safe to allow patients to stand with full weight-bearing at an early postoperative stage after submaximal resection of the sacrum, even if only half of S1 was preserved. This finding was supported by Simpson et al. (1995), who reported that no pelvic or spinal instability developed after a subtotal sacrectomy. In their series, an autogenous bone graft was used to restore the continuity of the pelvic ring in patients who had had a hemisacrectomy. A Four-strut graft was reported by Takahashi et al. (1983) after a subtotal sacrectomy in a patient with a huge giant cell tumor who lost stability between the lower lumbar column and the pelvis. They used the autogenous fibula as bilateral fore struts, and Harrington distraction rods as bilateral hind struts. This patient could walk without an external support nearly a year and a half postoperatively. The fore-strut fibula graft was inserted between the anterior portion of the vertebral body and the ilium. After a total sacrectomy, massive grafts from iliac bones and fibulae were inserted between the laminae, the transverse processes of the third and fourth lumbar vertebrae, and the iliac bones, together with Harrington distraction and compression rods (Shikita et al. 1988). After a total sacrectomy, Tomita and Tsuchiya (1990) reported that iliac bones and the autoclaved sacrum were grafted to fill up the dead space, and fibulae were fixed between the pedicle of the fourth lumbar vertebra and the iliac wing. The iliac wings, or a massive allograft, were used for a reconstruction by Sung et al. (1987). Posterior iliac flaps with their muscle attachments were mobilized behind the lower lumbar segment, and were supplemented with a sacral bar positioned between the bilateral iliac crests. The integrity of the pelvic ring was reestablished by fusion to the lower lumbar region posteriorly (Leung 1992).

In this series, sacral amputation was performed in seven patients. Because of the patients' ages and the short follow-up times, we could not fully assess their resulting bladder, bowel, and motor functions. Gennari et al. (1987) and Samson et al. (1993) discussed the relationship between the preserved sacral nerve-roots and sphincter control. Taking their results and ours together, and considering patients in whom the second sacral roots were the most caudad nerve-roots preserved, half of them had normal or nearly normal bladder and bowel control. However, patients in whom the most caudad roots preserved were the first sacral or more cephalic roots had impaired bladder and/or bowel control. Patients who had a unilateral resection of the sacrum, and in whom the most caudad roots preserved were the first sacral nerve and intact sacral nerves on the ipsilateral side, had a prompt recovery of sphincter function after surgery. Campanacci (1990) reported that sacrifice of the 4th and 5th sacral nerves bilaterally, and of the 3rd nerve on one side only, does not involve sphincter disorders, but (if the 3rd nerve is sacrificed on one side) results in perineal hypoesthesia alone.

Implants for Reconstruction

Various implants have been used in the reconstruction of defects resulting from resection of a pelvic bone tumor. In order to attach the lower lumbar spine to the pelvis, Harrington compression and distraction rods were used in cases 1, 2, and 3 of the Case Study section of this book. These rods proved to be effective in restoring the compressive and tensile loads encountered during gait. The Isola spinal system was useful for attachments extending from the lumbar spine, through the pelvis, to the lower extremities. This system used single or dual rods fixed with pedicle screws to L5 and S1, together with a transverse connector or Steffee plate with screws into the femur (Abumi 1996). A combination of sacral rods or AO plates with Harrington rods or the Cottrel–Dubousset system was also used (Tomita and Tsuchiya 1990). Various stainless steel plates and screws are available for the reconstruction of an interrupted pelvic ring, and for the immobilization of bone grafts.

Various endoprosthetic replacements, made of surgical stainless steel (316L), cobalt alloys, or titanium alloy, have been used for reconstructions after periacetabular resection. Abudu et al. (1997) reported a two-stage procedure in which a custom-made hemipelvic prosthesis was implanted after the temporary use of an acrylic resin construct and a conventional cemented femoral prosthesis. A conventional Stanmore femoral prosthesis with a 32-mm head was used in a one-stage procedure. Johnson (1978) implanted a Charnley–Mueller total hip replacement, and reconstituted the pelvic ring with cement reinforced by Küntscher rods and heavy Kirschner wires. Replacement with a cementless modular endoprosthesis and a composite of an allograft containing a long-stemmed cemented prosthesis has also been reported (Campanacci 1990).

Surgical Team

The operative treatment of a pelvic tumor is a complex, time-consuming, and often multistage procedure in both resection and reconstruction. It would be almost impossible for a single operative team to carry it out, and two or three teams are needed, all of whom fully know and understand the steps and sequences of the procedure. The members of such orthopedic teams should be skilled in spine and hip surgery, and the use of spinal instruments and endoprostheses. The operative team treating a pelvic tumor should include a general surgeon to take care of any anal or rectal problems, and a colostomy if one is needed, a urologist for urological problems, which very occasionally require an ileal conduit, a gynecologist for gynecological problems, a plastic surgeon for vascularized bone grafting and skin closure, and anesthesiologists for lengthy anesthesia and occasional massive bleeding. Furthermore, it is most important to have surgical nursing staff who know the procedures very well. Although the operation is a really challenging procedure, it is definitely worthwhile since the patient's quality of life can be greatly improved.

References

Abudu A, Grimer RJ, Cannon SR, Carter SR, Sneath RS (1997) Reconstruction of the hemipelvis after the excision of malignant tumors. Complications and functional outcome of prostheses. J Bone Joint Surg 79-B:773–779

Abumi K (1996) Reconstruction of the pelvic ring in cases of traumatic fracture and destruction due to bone tumor. OS NOW 22:198–207

Campanacci M (1990) Resection of the sacrum. Resection of the pelvis. Bone and soft-tissue tumors. Springer, Wien, New York, pp 59–66

Campanacci M (1999) Bone and soft tissue tumors. Clinical features, imaging, pathology and treatment. Piccin Nuova Libraria, Padova, and Springer, Wien, New York

Campanacci M, Capanna R (1991) Pelvic resections. The Rizzoli Institute experience. Orthop Clin N Am 22:65–86

Campanacci M, Guernelli N, Capanna R (1987) Pelvic resections involving and not involving the acetabulum. In: Coombs R, Friedlaender G (eds) Bone tumour management. Butterworths, London, pp 114–118

Carnesale PG (1998) General principles of tumors. In: Canale ST (ed) Campbell's operative othropaedics, 9th edn. Mosby, St. Louis, pp 643–682

Enneking WF (1983) Musculoskeletal tumor surgery. Churchill Livingston, New York, pp 483–529

Enneking WF, Dunham WK (1978) Resection and reconstruction for primary neoplasms involving the innominate bone. J Bone Joint Surg 60-A:731–746

Enneking WF, Menendez WK (1987) Functional evaluation of various reconstructions after periacetabular resection of iliac lesions. In: Enneking WF (ed) Limb salvage in musculoskeletal oncology. Churchill Livingstone, New York, pp 117–135

Enneking WF, Dunham W, Gebhardt MC, Malawar M, Pritchard DJ (1993) A system for the functional evaluation of reconstructive procedures after surgical treatment of tumors of the musculoskeletal system. Clin Orthop 286:241–246

Gennari L, Azzarelli A, Quagliuolo V (1987) A posterior approach for the excision of sacral chordoma. J Bone Joint Surg 69-B:565–568

Guest CB, Bell RA, Davis A, Langer F, Ling H, Gross AE, Czitrom A (1990) Allograft-implant composite reconstruction following periacetabular sarcoma resection. J Arthroplasty 5:S25–S34

Gunterberg B, Romanus B, Stener B (1976) Pelvic strength after major amputation of the sacrum. Acta Orthop Scand 47:635–642

Harrington KD (1981) The management of acetabular insufficiency secondary to metastatic malignant disease. J Bone Joint Surg 63-A:653–664

Harrington KD, Johnston JO, Kaufer HN, Luck JV, Moore TM (1986) Limb salvage and prosthetic joint reconstruction for low-grade and selected high-grade sarcomas of bone after wide resection and replacement by autoclaved autogenic grafts. Clin Orthop 211: 180–214

Heare TC, Enneking WF, Heare MM (1989) Staging techniques and biopsy of bone tumors. Orthop Clin North Am 20:273–285

Ilizarov GA (1992) Transosseous osteosynthesis. Theoretical and clinical aspects of the regeneration and growth of tissue. Springer, Berlin, Heidelberg

Johnson JTH (1978) Reconstruction of the pelvic ring following tumor resection. J Bone Joint Surg 60-A:747–751

Kusuzaki K, Shinjo H, Kim W, Nakamura S, Murata H, Hirasawa Y (1998) Resection hip arthroplasty for malignant pelvic tumor. Outcome in five patients followed more than 2 years. Acta Orthop Scand 69:617–621

Langlais F, Vielpeau C (1989) Allografts of the hemipelvis after tumor resection. J Bone Joint Surg 71-B:58–62

Leung PC (1992) Reconstruction of the pelvic ring after tumor resection. Int Orthop 16:168–171

Mnaymneth W, Lane J, Malinin TI, Glasser D (1997) Pelvic allografts in surgery of pelvic bone tumors. Chir Organi Mov 25:255–257

Nilsonne U, Kreicbergs A, Olsson E, Stark A (1982) Function after pelvic tumour resection involving the acetabular ring. Int Orthop (SICOT) 6:27–33

O'Connor MI, Sim FH (1989) Salvage of the limb in the treatment of malignant pelvic tumors. J Bone Joint Surg 71-A:481–494

O'Connor MI, Sim FH (1992) Pelvic tumors. In: Lewis MM (ed) Musculoskeletal oncology. A multidisciplinary approach. WB Saunders, Philadelphia, pp 253–264

Osaka S (1995) Surgical treatment of pelvic tumors. Toriyama S (ed) Kyorin Shoin, Tokyo

Osaka S, Toriyama S (1987) Surgical treatment of giant cell tumors of the pelvis. Clin Orthop 222:123–131

Rosenberg AG, Mankin HJ (1986) Complications of allograft surgery. In: Epps CH Jr (ed) Complications in orthopedic surgery, 2nd edn, vol 2. JB Lippincott, Philadelphia, pp 1385–1417

Samson IR, Springfield DS, Suit HD, Mankin HJ (1993) Operative treatment of sacrococcygeal chordoma. A review of twenty-one cases. J Bone Joint Surg 75-A:1476–1484

Sanjay BKS, Frassica FJ, Frassica DA, Unni KK, McLeod RA, Sim FH (1993) Treatment of giant-cell tumor of the pelvis. J Bone Joint Surg 75-A:1466–1475

Shikita J, Yamamuro T, Kotoura Y, Mikawa Y, Iida H, Maetani S (1988) Total sacrectomy and reconstruction for primary tumors. Report of two cases. J Bone Joint Surg 70-A:112–125

Simpson AHRW, Porter A, Davis A, Griffin A, McLeod RS, Bell RS (1995) Cephalad sacral resection with a combined extended ilioinguinal and posterior approach. J Bone Joint Surg 77-A:405–411

Steel HH (1978) Partial or complete resection of the hemipelvis. An alternative to hindquarter amputation for periacetabular chondrosarcoma of the pelvis. J Bone Joint Surg 60-A:719–730

Stener B, Gunterberg B (1978) High amputation of the sacrum for extirpation of tumors. Principles and technique. Spine 3:351–366

Sung HW, Shu WP, Wang HM, Yuai SY, Tsai YB (1987) Surgical treatment of primary tumors of the sacrum. Clin Orthop 215:91–98

Takahashi H, Tojo T, Morita T, Suzuki Y, Tajima T (1983) Treatment of sacral and sacroiliac tumors. J West Orthop Assoc, Abstr 3rd Congress Spinal Sect WPOA, pp 48–50

Tomita K, Tsuchiya H (1990) Total sacrectomy and reconstruction for huge sacral tumors. Spine 15:1223–1227

Uchida A, Myoui A, Araki N, Yoshikawa H, Ueda T, Aoki Y (1996) Prosthetic reconstruction for periacetabular malignant tumors. Clin Orthop 326:238–245

van der Lei B, Hoekstra HJ, Veth RPH, Ham SJ, Oldhoff J, Koops HS (1992) The use of the saddle prosthesis for reconstruction of the hip joint after tumor resection of the pelvis. J Surg Oncol 50:216–219

Yajima H, Tamai S, Mizzumoto S, Sugimura M, Horiuchi K (1992) Vascularized fibular graft for reconstruction after resection of aggressive benign and malignant bone tumors. Microsurgery 13:227–233

Microsurgical Reconstruction After Pelvic Tumor Resection

Minoru Shibata

Summary. The pelvis is the largest bone in the body. Various bone tumors may originate in the pelvis. The abundant circulation to the pelvic bones may be responsible, in part, for disseminating various types of metastatic tumors. In their early stages, these tumors may grow into the pelvic cavity without being noticed. Radical resection of these tumors frequently produces large and complex bone and soft-tissue defects.

An external hemipelvectomy, which requires the removal of a healthy lower limb below the hip, is not always well accepted by patients. However, an internal hemipelvectomy has to be followed by procedures to reconstruct the pelvic ring and hip joint in order to achieve a reasonably active postoperative lifestyle for these patients. Reconstructions using an allograft or an autoclaved autogenous bone graft may cause numerous complications associated with the presence of these large devascularized tissues. This problem may be avoided, and early union and stable gait may be achieved, by rebuilding the pelvic ring using microsurgical reconstruction with sections of dual or double-barreled free fibula. Filling a large defect with well-vascularized tissue and covering the defect with stable skin are crucial for the treatment of difficult infected wounds. A vascularized latissimus dorsi myocutaneous flap transfer with long vein grafts may serve as a useful tool in such difficult situations.

Key words. Microsurgery, Reconstruction, Tissue transfer, Pelvic tumor, Vein graft

Introduction

The pelvis is the largest bone in the body. The restoration of its continuity as a ring is important for the maintenance of weight transmission between the body trunk and the lower limbs. The trunk of the body is connected to the pelvis through the sacroiliac joint, and the pelvic ring transfers the weight of the upper body to the lower extremities through the hip joints.

Local aggressive tumors, such as a chordoma or chondrosarcoma, originate from the sacrum, and affect one or both sacroiliac joints. A wide or radical resection of these types of lesion may result in the disarticulation of one or both of these joints.

Wide resection of malignant tumors such as an Ewing's sarcoma may produce a large defect in the hemipelvic region. A hemipelvectomy, including ipsilateral total lower limb resection, has been the procedure of choice in this situation. An alternative procedure is based on the placement of an allograft or an autoclaved autogenous bone graft. However, significant complications resulting from the presence of large nonvascularized bone grafts are often encountered (Harrington 1992). Reconstruction using microsurgical tissue transfer of a large bone may represent a useful alternative option.

Irradiation of the pelvic area for a bone tumor, or for an invasive carcinoma of an internal pelvic organ, may occasionally lead to a difficult chronic ulcer. Local flap coverage of the irradiated ischemic fibrous tissue often fails to close these ulcers. It is also very difficult to locate appropriate recipient vessels around the ulcer for a vascularized tissue transfer. Long-vein grafting to an artery and vein may solve these recipient vessel problems (Nahai and Hagerty 1986; Salibian et al. 1983).

A team approach by tumor surgeons and microsurgeons is indispensable for appropriate surgical treatment of these difficult pelvic tumors. The tumor surgeon needs to be as objective as possible in order to obtain a safe surgical margin, and should not focus too much on how the resected tissues will be reconstructed. However, identification, gentle handling, and tagging of the stumps of important tissues such as neurovascular bundles or tendons, as well as preserving a safe margin approximately 5 mm long of ligated stumps of vessels for possible later vascular anastomosis, are extremely helpful in order that the microsurgeons can perform an efficient reconstruction. The microsurgeon has to be extremely careful to avoid postoperative vascular complications, since the failure of an important large tissue transfer may jeopardize the patient's life. Donor site morbidity needs to be as small as possible, and balanced with the relative merits obtained from the reconstruction methods available.

Based on meticulous preoperative planning and discussion between surgical teams, we performed novel and complicated tissue transfers to attain improved results in pelvic tumor surgery.

Reconstruction of a Large Bone Defect

Pelvic Ring Reconstruction

A chordoma is a rare neoplasm derived from embryonic remnants of the notochord, and arises mainly in the cranium and sacrococcygeal region. A sacrococcygeal chordoma grows slowly, widely infiltrates local tissues, and can metastasize, although metastasis is almost always late if it occurs at all. Resection of these tumors with a surrounding margin of normal tissue, using both anterior and posterior approaches, is recommended. These procedures occasionally fail to preserve a stable sacroiliac joint. A chondoma or chondrosarcoma in this area may require procedures similar to those for a chordoma.

Instrumentation for the Stabilization of One or Both Sacroiliac Joints

Fixation devices such as a sacral bar have been used to obtain stability and force transmission between the pelvis and the spinal column. This represents the simplest stabilization procedure for sacroiliac instability. However, loosening of this type of fixation is always a concern, especially in cases with bilateral sacroiliac joint instability.

Combination of Instrumentation and Free Vascularized Fibula Strut Grafting for a Sacroiliac Joint

A free vascularized fibula strut graft can be combined with a sacral bar to decrease the problem of loosening which is encountered when the sacral bar is used alone. The fibula is a long bone vascularized by the peroneal vessels. A fibular strut, a maximum of 28 cm long, can be elevated. The elevated fibula can be divided into two segments, forming a double-barreled flap. The fibula can also be divided into three segments so that an appropriate length of its central segment can be removed subperiosteally, thereby preserving the vascularization to the other two segments (Fig. 1). This technique provides the vascular freedom required for setting in the fibula struts to bridge the gap between the preserved sacrum and the lower lumbar vertebrae (Yajima and Tamai 1994).

Instrumentation Combined with Chain-Linked Free Flaps

It is well known that the peroneal artery is the vascular pedicle of the fibula, and is a flow-through system. Its distal end can serve as an excellent recipient artery for a second free flap. Using this technique, bilateral fibulae can be combined as a dual graft (Fig. 2), and even a third flap, such as a latissimus dorsi myocutaneous flap, can be connected for soft-tissue coverage (Figs. 3, 4). We believe that a combination of

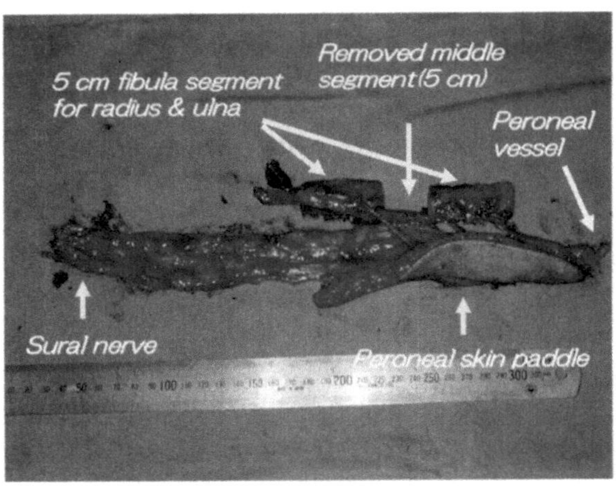

FIG. 1. A 15-cm section of fibula was elevated on the peroneal artery and vein, together with a skin paddle and the sural nerve. The elevated fibula was divided into three 5-cm-long segments. The center segment was removed subperiosteally to obtain more freedom to inset the other two segments

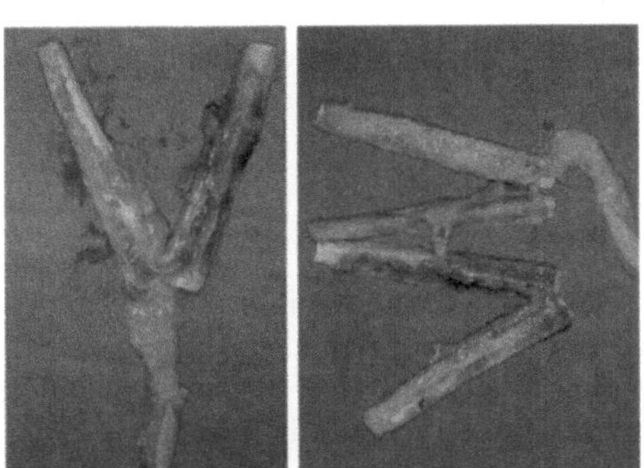

FIG. 2. *Left*, a double-barreled fibula graft with monitoring buoy flap. *Right*, the combination of a bilateral double-barreled fibula graft with vascular anastomosis between the peroneal vessels

FIG. 3. Diagram of combined chain-link-type flaps for a large and complex defect. The flap with the flow-through artery was used as the recipient artery for the second flap

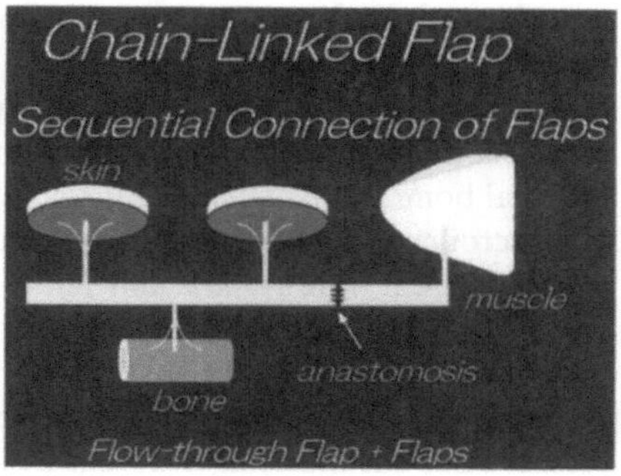

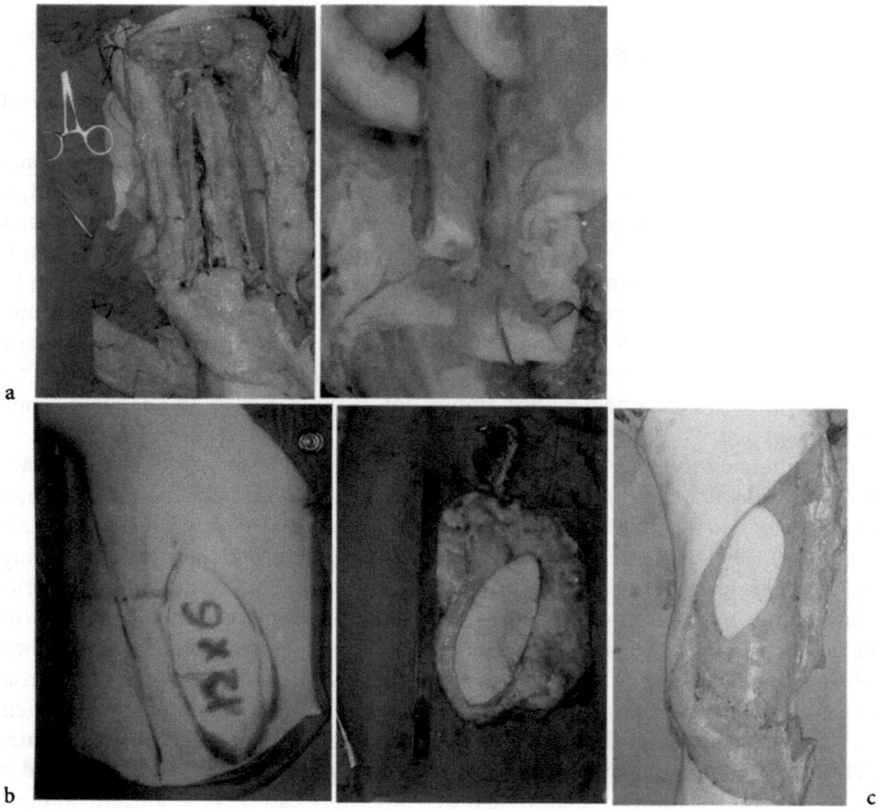

FIG. 4. **a** Dual fibula grafting combined with a Kuntcher nail for knee arthrodesis. The ipsilateral fibula was elevated as a pedicled flap, and turned up into the defect. The distal ends of the peroneal vessels of the pedicled fibula were connected to those of the contralateral free fibula. The distal end of the free fibula demonstrated good bleeding after vascular anastomosis. **b** A latissimus dorsi myocutaneous flap was elevated. **c** The latissimus dorsi muscle was placed on the dual fibula graft and revascularized by anastomosis of the thoracodorsal vessels to the distal peroneal vessels of the free fibula graft

vascularized fibula and instrumentation is a useful method for the stabilization of the pelvis to the spinal column.

Reconstruction of a unilateral sacroiliac joint allows a different approach to be used, such as double-barreled fibula grafting combined with the application of an external bone fixator, since the instability is much less than that resulting from bilateral sacroiliac resection. The double-barreled fibula grafting method can fill a defect less than 13 cm wide (Yajima and Tamai 1994), while the dual fibula grafting technique will allow reconstruction of wider defects up to 28 cm. There have been no reports in the literature on the dual fibula bone grafting method for pelvic ring reconstruction. However, this procedure seems to be very feasible based on our experience of a successful knee fusion using a 28-cm dual fibula bone graft, and of bridging a 14-cm defect in the femoral metaphysis using a dual double-barreled fibula graft. Yajima and Tamai (1994) reported that if union is achieved, hypertrophic changes of the fibula can be expected, which will reflect the adjustment of the fibula to the different mechanical environment.

Reconstruction After Internal Hemipelvectomy

The best surgical approach for resection of Ewing's sarcoma remains controversial (Scully et al. 1995). A wide resection of Ewing's sarcoma may require excision of the hemipelvis, including the hip joint, resulting a massive and extremely complicated defect. Reconstruction of this type of defect may be performed using an allograft, or an autoclaved or extracorporeally irradiated autograft (Harrington 1992). However, it is difficult for such large bone grafts to become revascularized, and easy for them to become infected or fractured. At the present time, only a reconstruction using an autogenous tissue graft can circumvent the problems mentioned above. A widely accepted treatment for this type of malignant tumor is an external hemipelvectomy, which is often very difficult for the patient to accept. It is well known that the function of the lower extremity after a below-knee amputation is quite high if an adequate simple brace is applied.

We amputated the lower limb of a patient with Ewing's sarcoma of the ilium at a level below the knee, and used portions of the amputated limb for reconstruction, as described in detail by Saito in chapter 6. This procedure is now briefly summarized (Fig. 5a–e). The amputated foot was used for the reconstruction of the pelvic ring, and the ankle joint was used to reconstruct the hip joint. Both posterior and anterior tibial arteries were anastomosed for revascularization. Bony union was attained with the opposite pubic bone anteriorly and with the sacrum posteriorly. The patient was able to ambulate with a crutch 6 months after surgery. However, the patient died from lung metastases of the original tumor. This procedure was applied to another patient with Ewing's sarcoma of the pelvis. Unfortunately, the second patient died from lung metastases before ambulation. However, successful tissue transfer was confirmed at the time of the autopsy. We believe that this procedure can serve as a useful alternative reconstructive technique for patients for whom an external hemipelvectomy is indicated.

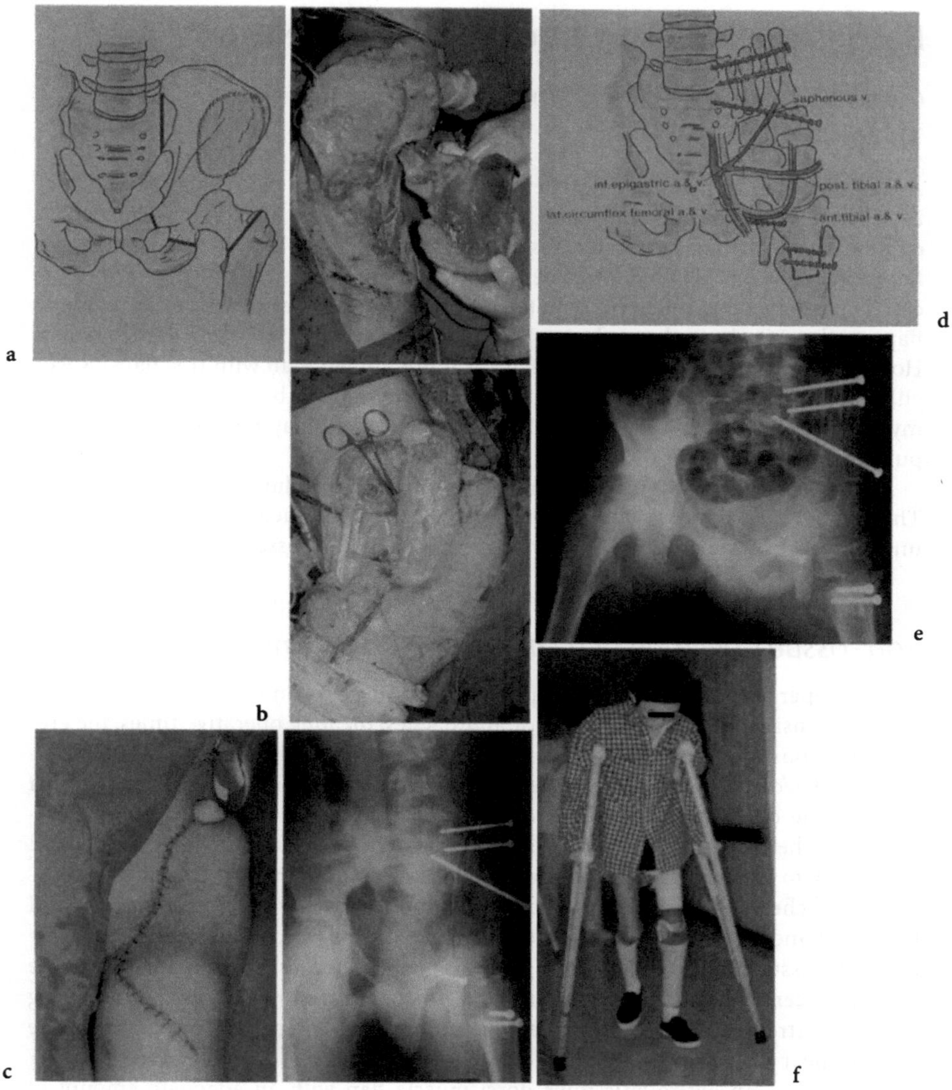

FIG. 5. **a** An internal hemipelvectomy was performed. **b** Below-knee amputation on the left side was carried out. The foot and ankle were grafted into the defect (See Fig. 7, page 93). **c** The completed surgery. The monitoring toe pulp was later removed. The foot was used for pelvic ring reconstruction, and the ankle for hip joint reconstruction. **d** Schematic diagram showing the procedure. Two sets of arteries and veins were repaired. **e** Four months after surgery. Bone union was complete. **f** The patient could walk using a crutch. At this point, there was 60° flexion, 20° extension, 10° abduction, and 10° adduction in the reconstructed left hip joint

Reconstruction of a Large Soft-Tissue Defect

Coverage Using Pedicled Flaps and a Free Split Thickness Skin Graft

A local skin flap with a random pattern of vascular supply is not reliable when raised in a large size. However, an axial pattern flap based on an adipofascial pedicle containing cutaneous perforator vessels, such as a gluteal artery-based perforator flap, may safely be extended into a defect of considerable size. A large flap of this size can be partially de-epithelized to fill the defect. A gluteal artery-based myocutaneous flap can be raised as a large flap, as well as a tensor fascia lata myocutaneous flap. However, the freedom to inset these flaps is more limited than with free flaps. A vascular pedicled flap, such as a deep inferior epigastric artery-based rectus abdominus myocutaneous flap obtained from the upper abdomen, may be used for a similar purpose.

A split-thickness skin graft is a simpler alternative procedure for wound coverage. This type of graft requires careful wound care, that is continued after tumor resection until the base of the defect is filled with clean granulation tissue.

Soft-Tissue Coverage of a Large Infected Wound

The postoperative infection rate for pelvic tumor surgery can be high because of the use of extensive anterior and posterior approaches, the long operative times, the creation of a postoperative defect with a large dead space, and the use of instrumentation for defect stabilization. Repeated curettage and irrigation of the infected area through the open wound is often required to cure these difficult infections. Postoperative thermotherapy by warm saline irrigation or irradiation may be applied repeatedly to secure tumor eradication. All of these procedures may result in the formation of chronic wide ulcers. A sufficient amount of well-vascularized tissue to fill the defect and cover the wound is necessary to make the infection settle down. A vascularized tissue transfer is demanding for this purpose because the surrounding tissue is tightly scarred by the intraoperative and postoperative procedures. This scarring makes it extremely difficult to prepare adequate, reliable recipient vessels for tissue transfer near the wound.

We selected an entire latissimus dorsi muscle flap with an adequate amount of skin for the tissue transfer. This flap is one of the most reliable flaps because the thoracodorsal artery and vein, which serve as the vascular pedicle, both have a large diameter. We elongated the thoracodorsal artery and vein by placing long interpositioning grafts from the small saphenous vein.

The surgical team is divided into two groups. One group elevates the latissimus dorsi flap, and the other group performs curettage and preparation of the recipient wound, and elevation of the small saphenous vein bilaterally.

A skin flap of sufficient size to cover the wound is designed over the latissimus dorsi muscle, and dissection is initiated from its anterior site. The thoracodorsal vessels are carefully identified and protected from injury. The origin of the flap is severed, and the flap is elevated on its vascular pedicle. However, the insertion of the flap is left attached. A subcutaneous tunnel is made through the incision for flap dissection and to the recipient wound for later transfer of the flap with the elongated vascular pedicle. A section of the small saphenous vein, approximately 33 cm long, is harvested from both limbs. The saphenous vein graft is interposed in the proximal portion of the thoracodorsal artery in an up-side-down position, taking care to not rotate the graft. There may be a discrepancy between the diameters of the suturing vessels. An oblique or fish-mouth cut of the suturing vessel stumps may be helpful to adjust the diameters. The other small saphenous vein is interposed in the proximal thoracodorsal vein in an upright position without rotation. After releasing the vascular clamps, circulation to the flap is confirmed and the distal insertion of the latissimus muscle is then detached. The flap, based solely on the elongated vascular pedicle, is brought into the subcutaneous tunnel and pulled out into the recipient site. The wound is closed in layers with suction drainage.

We have used this procedure for four patients with an infected large defect surrounded by cicatricial tissue. All flaps were successfully transferred without partial necrosis, and the deep infections eventually subsided.

Case Presentations

Case 1. 57-Year-Old Man with Chondrosarcoma of the Sacrum

Preoperative X-ray films and computed tomography identified an 8 cm × 10 cm tumor originating from the sacrum and protruding into the internal pelvis (Fig. 6a–c). The patient experienced a lower leg palsy and vesicorectal disturbance. A staged operation for tumor removal was planned. A colostomy and the setting of an artificial anus, and ligation of the internal iliac artery were initially performed in preparation for the following staged surgery for tumor resection. Three months after the first operation, a second procedure for tumor resection was performed using anterior and posterior approaches. The tumor was removed by resecting the sacrum with the fifth lumbar vertebra. The spinal column was stabilized using a sacral bar (Fig. 6d). Postoperative pathologic examination of the tumor identified chondrosarcoma. However, a deep infection developed postoperatively. Fourteen months after the first surgery, debridement was performed and resulted in a massive 18 cm × 25 cm defect (Fig. 6e). The wound was closed using a latissimus dorsi myocutaneous flap. Scars made by the local flap elevation and the ligation of the internal iliac artery at the first operation, as well as scar formation resulting from the extensive dissection of the tumor, made the preparation of the recipient vessels for flap transfer extremely difficult. A latissimus dorsi flap was transferred by elongating its vascular pedicle using long vein grafts. The procedure is represented schematically in Fig. 6f. The wound was closed successfully (Fig. 6g), and controllable recurrences of the wound infection were noted postoperatively. The sacral bar instruments were eventually removed in order to control the infection. At the present time, there is no evidence of wound infection, and the patient can remain in the sitting position without difficulty for a

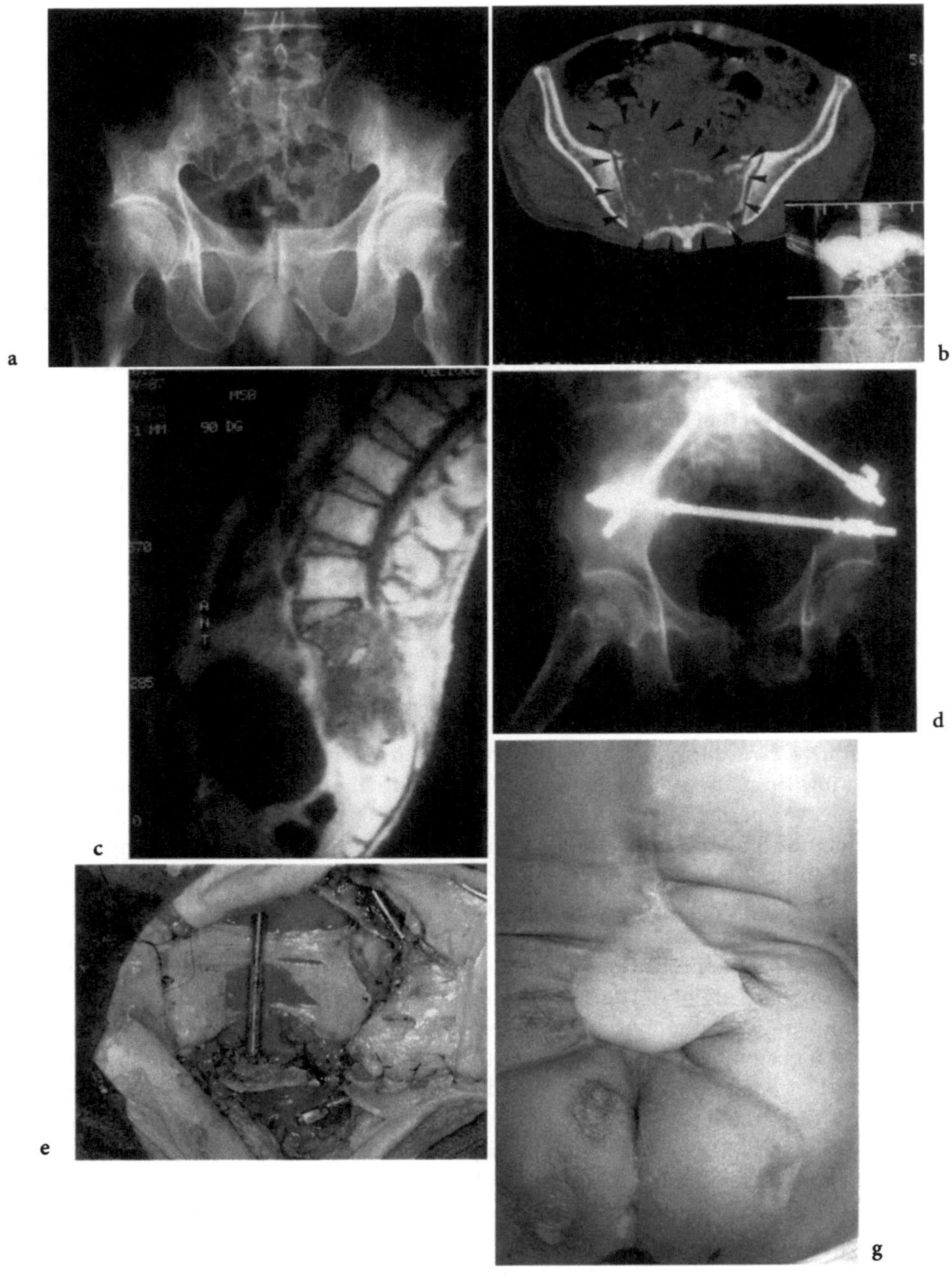

FIG. 6. **a** Anterior–posterior X-ray view showing a sacral bone tumor. **b** Computed tomography of the sacral area. The sacrum had been destroyed, and the tumor was protruding into the internal pelvic area. **c** Longitudinal section by computed tomography. The tumor was growing anteriorly, compressing the bladder. **d** A sacral bar was placed for stabilization. **e** After debridement of the infected wound. **f** Schematic diagram of the latissimus dorsi myocutaneous flap transfer using long vein grafts. **g** The wound was successfully closed by the flap

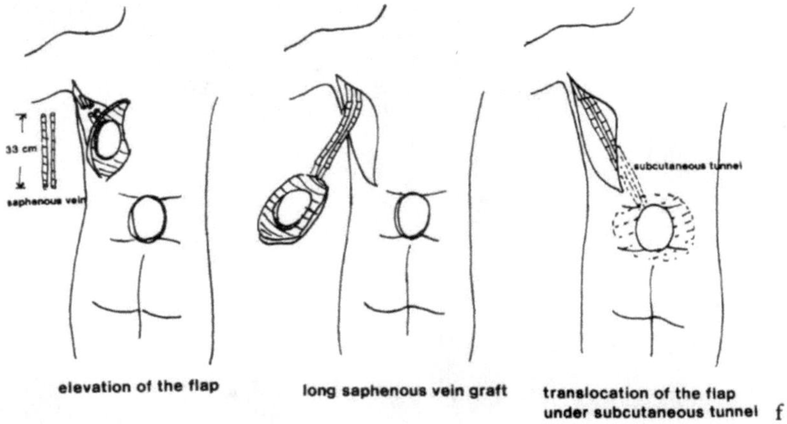

FIG. 6. *Continued*

considerable period of time, in spite of a nonunion between the spinal column and the ilium. (See Chapter 10, Case 17, p 185)

Case 2. 58-Year-Old Woman with Closure of a Deep Infected Chronic Ulcer in the Sacral Area

A large portion of the sacrum was defective, and sclerotic dead bone was partially exposed (Fig. 7a). The patient had previously undergone a hysterectomy and postoperative irradiation to the internal pelvic area at the age of 38. She had undergone several operations before presenting to our clinic. Preoperative angiography identified severe left-side dominant vascular changes, such as sclerosis and stenosis associated with soft-tissue fibrosis, from the previous postoperative irradiation of the pelvic area (Fig. 7b). There were scars created by the elevation of the local flaps. Preoperative evaluation excluded the possibility of preparing adequate recipient vessels around the wound. Intensive wound care and systemic administration of vancomycin was performed preoperatively, and wound closure using a free latissimus dorsi myocutaneous flap was planned. Careful debridement was performed, taking care to not open the retroperitoneal space (Fig. 7c). The entire left latissimus dorsi muscle was elevated on the thoracodorsal vessels, except at the muscle's insertion (Fig. 7d). The harvested small saphenous veins were interposed in the thoracodorsal vessels in order to obtain the necessary elongation (Fig. 7e). Excellent perfusion to the flap was noted, and the latissimus dorsi muscle was then detached from its insertion for transfer into the sacral wound (Fig. 7f). The wound was closed in layers. The entire flap survived, and the infection subsided (Fig. 7g).

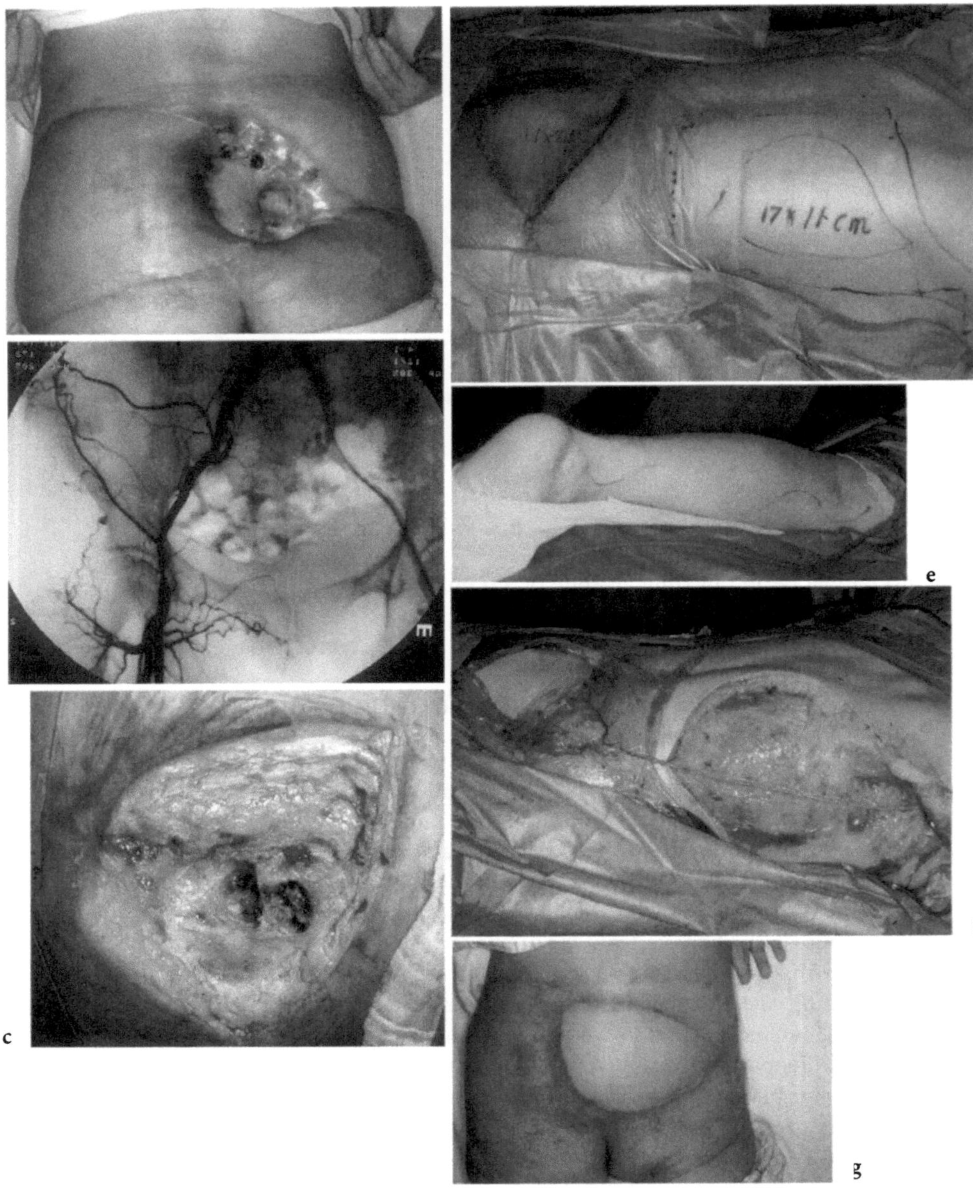

FIG. 7. **a** Preoperative condition. A deep infected wound with exposed sacral bone. **b** Angiogram showing the vascular changes associated with postoperative irradiation. The right iliac arterial system was markedly affected. **c** After debridement of the wound. **d** The design for latissimus dorsi myocutaneous flap elevation. **e** Bilateral small saphenous veins were harvested for grafting. **f** Vein grafts were interposed in the thoracodorsal artery and vein. Thoracodorsal vessel elongation allowed transfer of the latissimus dorsi flap into the sacral wound. **g** Successful transfer of the flap, and wound closure

References

Harrington KD (1992) The use of hemipelvic allografts or autoclaved grafts for reconstruction after wide resections of malignant tumors of the pelvis. J Bone Joint Surg 74-A:331–341
Nahai F, Hagerty R (1986) One-stage microvascular transfer of a latissimus flap to the sacrum using vein grafts. Plast Reconstr Surg 77:312–315
Salibian AH, Tesoro VR, Wood DL (1983) Staged transfer of a free microvascular latissimus dorsi myocutaneous flap using saphenous vein grafts. Plast Reconstr Surg 71:543–547
Scully SP, Temple HT, O'Keefe RJ, Scarborough MT, Mankin HJ, Gebhardt MC (1995) Role of surgical resection in pelvic Ewing's sarcoma. J Clin Oncol 13:2336–2341
Shibata M, Saito H, Seki T, Kinto N, Takahashi Y, Maruyama T (1990) A case with reconstruction of pelvic ring and hip joint using ipsilateral vascularized foot and ankle after wide resection of Ewing's tumor of the pelvis. J Jpn S R M 3:18–21
Yajima H, Tamai S (1994) Twin-barreled vascularized fibular grafting to the pelvis and lower extremity. Clin Orthop 303:178–184

Simultaneous Reconstruction of the Ilium and Hip Joint with a Free Vascularized Foot–Ankle Joint Graft After Wide Resection of Ewing's Sarcoma of the Ilium

HIDEHIKO SAITO

Summary. A 13-year-old boy with Ewing's sarcoma affecting the left iliac wing and the acetabular roof underwent an extensive internal hemipelvectomy and reconstruction with a vascularized foot–ankle joint graft harvested from the ipsilateral lower limb. He became ambulatory with a below-knee prosthesis, and obtained approximately 60° flexion and 5° abduction in the reconstructed hip joint. It was concluded that this procedure is a viable option for the reconstruction of a large defect created by an extensive internal hemipelvectomy which included the hip joint.

Key words. Ewing's sarcoma, Type II, Hip joint reconstruction, Free osteoarticular graft, Internal hemipelvectomy

Introduction

A large defect resulting from resection of the iliac wing can be reconstructed in several different ways, including the use of an allograft, a free vascularized or nonvascularized fibular graft, or a custom implant. A hindquarter amputation is a common treatment option when a tumorous lesion involves both the hip joint and the iliac wing. However, it seems irrational to sacrifice the entire intact portion of the lower limb below the hip joint with this approach. Limb salvage is very challenging in such a case because the defect created by excision of the tumor is very large. Methods for simultaneously reconstructing the pelvis and hip joint are limited, and include the use of an allograft, replacement with a customized hip joint prosthesis with a long stem (Uchida et al. 1992, 1996), or rotationplasty for the hip joint (Winkelmann 1986). The use of an allograft was not an option in Japan because it was illegal to harvest any organs except the kidney and cornea from a deceased individual until October 16, 1997, when the Law of Organ Transplantation was enacted.

A procedure was developed which provided for the simultaneous reconstruction of the iliac wing and the hip joint using a free vascularized foot–ankle joint graft harvested from the ipsilateral lower limb. This surgical technique is presented and discussed in the context of a case report.

Case History

A 13-year-old boy first experienced a fever and noted pain in his left buttock at the end of November 1988. The pain persisted, and swelling appeared soon thereafter. An X-ray examination at a local hospital revealed a lytic lesion in the left ilium. The patient was referred to the Niigata University Hospital on December 20 with suspicion of a malignant bone tumor. An 8 cm × 11 cm mass was palpated in the anterior portion of the ilium, and an 8.5 cm × 9.5 cm mass was palpated in the posterior portion of the ilium.

Radiographs showed a moth-eaten appearance in the anterior half of the left ilium, which extended to the acetabular roof (Fig. 1). Magnetic resonance imaging revealed a large tumorous mass involving the left ilium (Fig. 2a). The mass appeared to be growing both inside and outside the pelvic cavity. An angiogram revealed hyper-

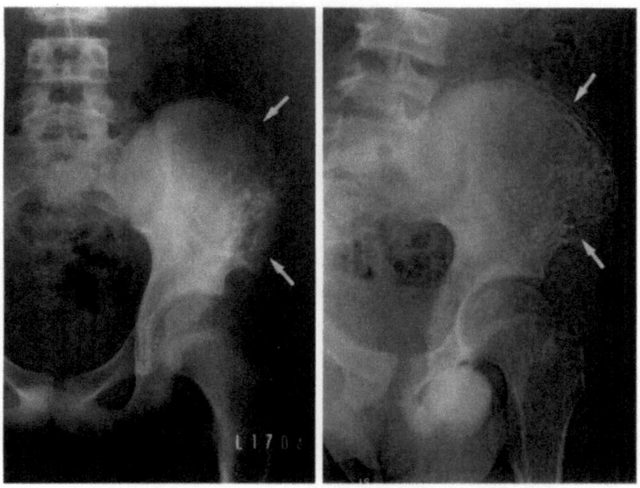

a b

FIG. 1a,b. Radiographs taken before chemotherapy and radiation therapy. **a** Anterior–posterior view of the left half of the pelvis. **b** Iliac wing view. *Arrows*, the boundary of the tumor

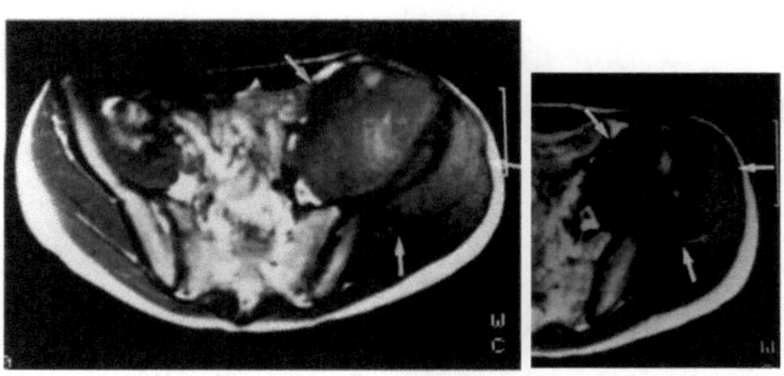

a b

FIG. 2. Magnetic resonance images **a** before and **b** after chemotherapy and radiation therapy. *Arrows*, the boundary of the tumor

vascularity in the anterior half of the ilium which extended along the posterior portion of the iliac crest (Fig. 3).

The following laboratory data were obtained: erythrocyte sedimentation rates of 76 mm/1 h and 118 mm/2 h; white blood cell count of $8700/mm^3$; lactic dehydrogenase of 1059 IU/l; alkaline phosphatase of 468 IU/l. The pathological findings of a specimen taken by a needle biopsy were compatible with Ewing's sarcoma (Fig. 4).

The patient received chemotherapy with the Rosen T-11 protocol (Rosen 1982) from January 10 to February 6, 1989, and also underwent radiation therapy from February 6 to 27, with a total of 3000 rads (Fig. 2b).

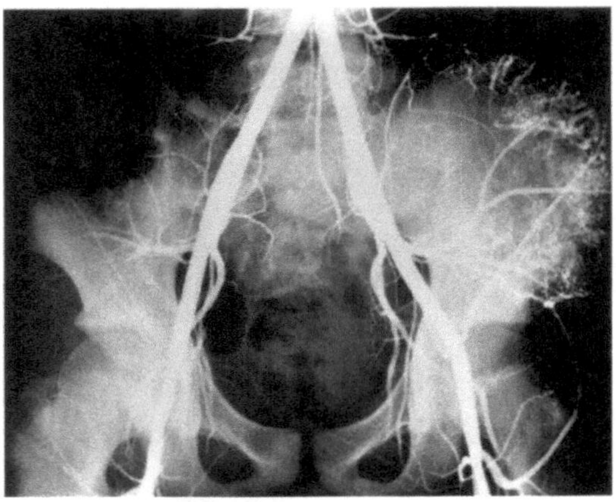

FIG. 3. Angiogram taken before chemotherapy and radiation therapy

a

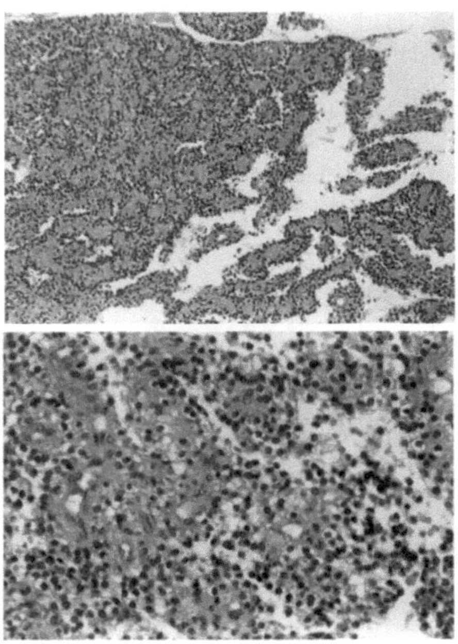

b

FIG. 4a,b. Photomicrographs of a specimen taken by a needle biopsy. **a** Low magnification (×25). **b** High magnification (×100)

On March 8, the patient underwent wide excision of the tumor, including the entire ilium and hip joint (extensive internal hemipelvectomy), and those were reconstructed simultaneously with a free vascularized foot–ankle joint graft using the distal portion of his own left lower extremity.

Operative Procedures

Wide Excision of the Tumor

A long skin incision was made in the abdominal wall along a line a few centimeters medial to the iliac crest. The proximal end of the incision was extended posteriorly along the posterior portion of the iliac crest, and the distal end of the incision was extended medially along the inguinal ligament (Fig. 5a). The retroperitoneal space was then entered by dividing the abdominal muscles along a line 3 cm from their attachment to the iliac crest, and then retracting them medially. The sartorius muscle and the lateral femoral cutaneous nerve were transected a few centimeters from the anterior superior iliac spine. The psoas muscle was dissected distally to the level of its tendinous portion, and was incised in a z-fashion (Fig. 5b). The external iliac artery and vein were exposed and protected. The iliacus muscle was transected at the level of the hip joint. The rectus femoris muscle was transected a few centimeters distal to its origin on the anterior inferior iliac spine. The superior ramus of the pubis was then exposed by dividing the origin of the pectineus muscle. The iliolumbar and lumbar arteries were identified and divided posteriorly in the retroperitoneal space (Fig. 5c). The iliolumbar ligament was divided, and the anterior aspect of the sacral wing was prepared for osteotomy. The quadratus lumborum muscle was transected at a level 3 cm cranial to the iliac crest.

The patient was then placed in a semiprone position. The proximal end of the operative incision was extended posteriorly along the iliac crest, and then curved caudally to the level of the sciatic notch (Fig. 6a). The distal end of the operative incision in the groin was further extended distally and posteriorly in the thigh (Figs. 5a, 6a). The posterior skin flap was dissected subcutaneously to the level of the anterior border of the gluteus maximus muscle. The flap was then elevated with the attached gluteus maximus by dividing the origin of the gluteus maximus 3 cm away from the iliac crest, and dissecting it off the underlying gluteus medius muscle. The musculocutaneous flap was reflected posteriorly by partially dividing its tendinous insertion (Fig. 6b). The branches of the superior gluteal artery, vein, and nerve passing into the gluteus medius and minimus muscles were divided. The insertions of the gluteus medius, gluteus minimus, and piriformis muscles were divided. The femoral neck was osteotomized. The posterior aspect of the sacroiliac joint was exposed by dissecting the sacrospinalis muscle off the ilium. An osteotomy was made in the sacrum medial to the joint, and was extended halfway anteriorly. The ischium was exposed by dividing the gemellus and obturator internus muscles, and was osteotomized at a level caudal to the acetabulum.

The patient was then placed in a semisupine position, and an osteotome was inserted posteriorly through the sacral wing to complete the osteotomy. The internal

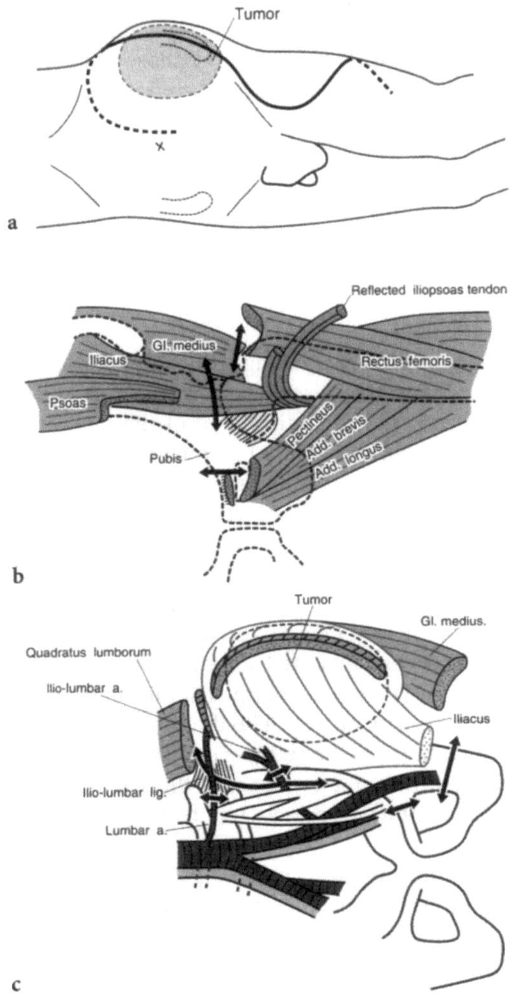

FIG. 5a–c. Operative procedures by the anterior approach. **a** Skin incision. **b** Procedures involving the muscles in the inguinal region. **c** Procedures in the retroperitoneal space of the pelvis

hemipelvectomy was completed by dividing the levator ani muscle and sacrospinous ligament while the ilium was being pulled outward.

Preparation of the Graft

A graft of the foot–ankle joint was harvested by amputating the ipsilateral leg through its distal fourth (Fig. 7). The graft was denuded of skin, and prepared by preserving three vascular pedicles: the dorsalis pedis artery and veins, the posterior tibial artery and veins, and the greater saphenous vein. All toes were amputated through the metatarsophalangeal joints. The pulp of the great toe, attached to the vascular pedicle of the dorsalis pedis artery and veins, was used as a monitor flap. The fifth metatarsal was osteotomized obliquely so that it would match the cut surface of the sacrum. The first and second metatarsals were shortened. The tibia was thinned so that it could be

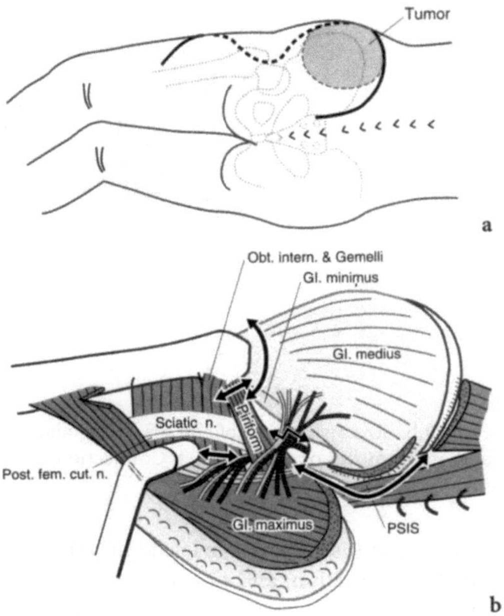

FIG. 6a,b. Operative procedures by the posterior approach. **a** Skin incision. **b** Procedures after the elevation of the gluteal musculocutaneous flap

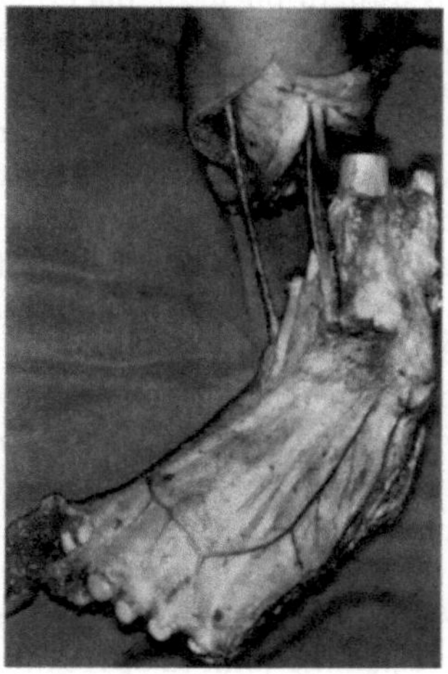

FIG. 7. Preparation of the graft consisting of the ipsilateral foot–ankle joint with vascular pedicles

inserted into the intramedullary canal of the proximal femur, which had been reosteotomized at the level of the intertrochanteric line. The medial aspect of the tuber calcanei was fashioned to accept the stump of the osteotomized ischium.

Reconstruction

After the graft was prepared, it was placed into the cavity created by the internal hemipelvectomy (Fig. 8a). The fifth metatarsal was fixed to the sacrum with three

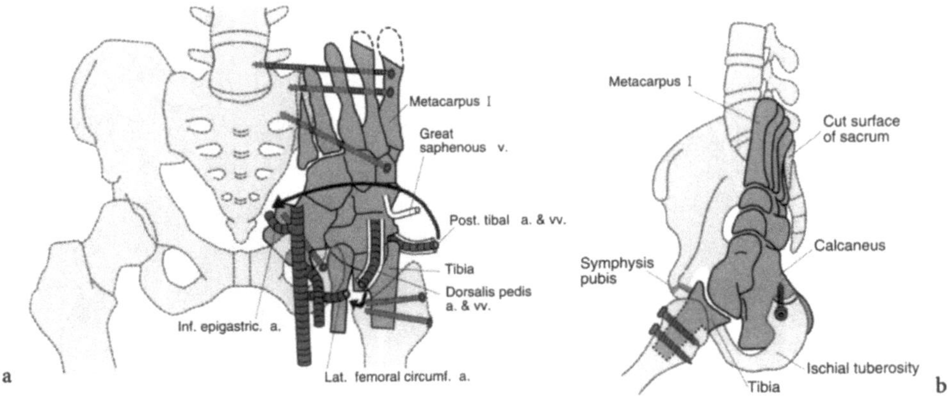

FIG. 8a,b. Reconstruction of the iliac wing and hip joint. **a** Fixation of the graft in the pelvis and anastomoses of the vessels. **b** Connection of the calcaneus and ischium

screws, and the tibia was inserted into the proximal femur and fixed with two screws. Finally, the ischium and calcaneus were connected with a screw (Fig. 8b). While performing these procedures, the sciatic nerve had to be translocated into the obturator foramen to avoid compression with the calcaneus. After completion of the internal fixation of the graft, the range of motion of the newly formed hip joint was assessed with gentle passive motion, revealing approximately 60° flexion, 30° extension, and 10° abduction.

The vascular pedicles were anastomosed to the recipient vessels with microsurgical techniques (Fig. 8a), the dorsalis pedis artery and veins to the lateral femoral circumflex artery and veins, the posterior tibial artery and veins to the inferior epigastric artery and veins, and the great saphenous vein to a vein in the adjacent area.

The quadratus lumborum muscle was first sutured to the tips of the metatarsals. The ends of the psoas tendon, which had been divided in a z-fashion, were sutured back together. The abdominal muscles were sutured to the periosteum of the first metatarsal, as was the anterior border of the gluteus maximus muscle of the posterior flap. The proximal border of the gluteus maximus was sutured to the quadratus lumborum muscle.

Two thick suction drains were placed, one anterior and one posterior to the graft. After putting on a sterile dressing, a long hip spica cast was applied with the newly created hip joint in approximately 40° flexion.

Postoperative Course

The operative wound healed after débridement of marginal wound necrosis and secondary skin closure. The patient resumed chemotherapy after recovery from the surgical intervention. The reconstructed hip joint was immobilized by the hip spica cast for 2 months. A radiograph taken 3 months after the operation showed that the transplanted foot between the sacrum and the proximal femur was stable (Fig. 9). The patient began walking exercises with a below-knee prosthesis 3 months after the

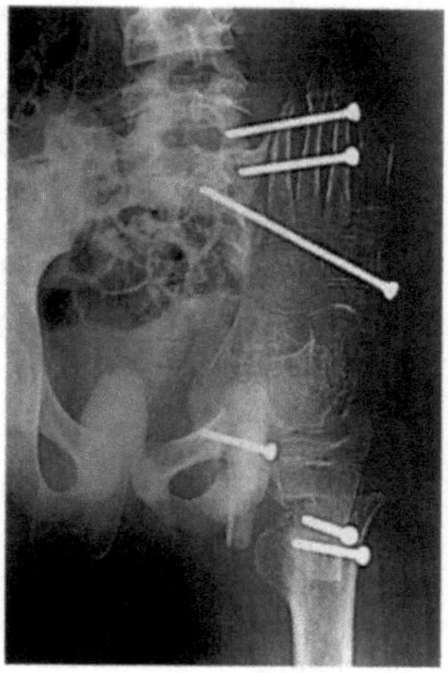

FIG. 9. Radiograph taken 3 months after the reconstruction procedure

surgical procedure. He was able to climb up and down stairs with one-third weight-bearing on the salvaged lower limb.

Tomography of the lung taken on May 9, 1989, 2 months after the operation, showed a metastatic lesion, 1 cm in diameter, in the upper lobe of the lungs bilaterally. The patient was again given chemotherapy, and then underwent a partial lobectomy on August 15.

Laminectomy of the second to fifth lumbar vertebrae was performed on December 10 because of spine metastasis.

The patient died of metastatic disease on March 2, 1990.

Discussion

Because of recent advances in chemotherapy and surgical techniques, internal hemipelvectomy has become a practical way to manage malignant tumors of the pelvis. There are four methods of functional reconstruction after internal hemipelvectomy: endoprosthesis, allograft, vascularized fibular graft, and hip rotationplasty.

Enneking (1983) proposed three major types of pelvic excision related to the three anatomical divisions of the innominate bone: iliac, periacetabular, and ischiopubic. Methods of management after excision of each division of the pelvis were described. Iliac and periacetabular divisions were excised in the case just presented. There are a limited number of ways to reconstruct the pelvis and hip joint simultaneously in such a situation.

Various types of customized endoprostheses have been used with reconstruction after an internal hemipelvectomy. However, the potential liabilities of this approach include loosening of the prosthesis and deep infection. The larger the pelvic defect, the higher the incidence of these complications. Hip rotationplasty is indicated for cases where the tumor involves the proximal femur. The knee joint serves as the hip joint in this procedure. Although a hip rotationplasty could be used in cases such as the one presented in this chapter by fixing the proximal stump of the femur to the sacrum, the absence of lateral movement in the reconstructed joint is a drawback, as well as the poor cosmetic appearance of the reconstruction.

Reconstruction with an allograft was not chosen for the patient presented in this chapter because at the time it was illegal to harvest any organs from a deceased individual except the kidney and cornea. In addition, it did not seem feasible to reconstruct a mobile hip joint with an allograft. Furthermore, it was felt that a vascularized fibular graft would be too small to fill the large defect created by an extensive internal hemipelvectomy.

Potential methods for the reconstruction of both the pelvis and the hip joint with a viable autograft were investigated. It was thought that the use of the distal portion of the ipsilateral limb, which would be discarded after a hindquarter amputation, would be an acceptable option. It is known that the functional outcome of a below-knee amputation is very good. Because of this, amputation through the distal leg to harvest a vascularized foot-ankle joint graft seemed justified.

The advantages of reconstruction with a vascularized foot-ankle joint graft are listed below.

1. The procedure provides a sufficient amount of bone to fill a large skeletal defect.
2. The total range of dorsiflexion–plantar flexion of the ankle joint is approximately 70°, which provides an adequate amount of flexion–extension for the reconstructed hip. In addition, varus–valgus motion at the ankle provides some hip adduction–abduction.
3. The calcaneus serves as the sciatic tuberosity, and provides stability in sitting.
4. A vascularized graft provides sufficient vascularity to the reconstructed region for the prevention of deep infection.

References

Enneking WF (1983) Musculoskeletal tumor surgery. Churchill Livingstone, New York, pp 494–522

Rosen G (1982) Current management of Ewing's sarcoma. Prog Clin Cancer 8:267–282

Uchida A, Shinto Y, Kudawara I, Yoshikawa H, Ono K, Ueda T, Hamada H (1992) A limb-saving operation for cases with malignant pelvic bone tumors. In: Uchida A, Ono K (eds) Recent advances in musculoskeletal oncology. Springer, Tokyo, pp 147–154

Uchida A, Myoui A, Araki N, Yoshikawa H, Ueda T, Aoki Y (1996) Prosthetic reconstruction for periacetabular malignant tumors. Clin Orthop 326:238–245

Winkelmann WW (1986) Hip rotationplasty for malignant tumors of the proximal part of the femur. J Bone Joint Surg Am 68:362–369

Chapter 7
Related Topics

Topics Relating to Pregnancy, Reconstruction, Vesicorectal Disturbance, and Complications

Tetsuo Hotta and Tetsuro Morita

Summary. Eight special topics relating to pregnancy, complications, the quality of life of the patient, and unique measures of reconstruction are introduced. Our experiences of the reconstruction of the external iliac vein using a crossover venous bypass, iliolumbar fusion after sacrectomy, and special reconstruction of the hip joint using a free osteoarticular ankle graft may be helpful for tumor surgeons facing similar difficulties. Some actual case reports are included in other chapters.

Key words. Pregnancy after hemipelvectomy, Crossover venous bypass, Reconstruction after sacrectomy, Herniation of the bowel, Reconstruction of the hip joint

Pregnancy and Normal Delivery After Hemipelvectomy

We treated a patient who became pregnant after a hemipelvectomy, and had a normal delivery. This case is described in Case 16 in Chap. 10, by A. Ogose, this volume. Similar cases are reported in the literature (Bergh et al. 1988; Holzaepfel 1973; Nuss and Lee 1967; Snyder and Thomas 1989; Stavrakas and Sanders 1983).

Reconstruction of Venous Drainage After Sacrificing the External Iliac Vein

We had a difficult case involving a patient with a malignant soft tissue tumor arising in the retroperitoneum. The external iliac artery and vein were involved in the tumor. The artery was reconstructed with an artificial vessel. In general, maintenance of the patency of artificial venous grafts is felt to be difficult. We created a crossover bypass graft of the greater saphenous vein to the affected distal stump of the greater saphenous vein. The details of this procedure are described in Case 13 in Chap. 10, by T. Hotta, this volume.

Reconstruction of the Sacroiliac Joint After Total Sacrectomy

Total sacrectomy may be the most difficult procedure encountered in pelvic surgery. Although resection of the entire sacrum is extremely difficult, its reconstruction is even more difficult. Sacral reconstruction involves many potential problems, such as the choice of graft materials and internal fixation devices, the control of infection, and the timing of the reconstruction, i.e., a one-stage procedure or a staged operation.

There is no gold standard for reconstruction of the sacrum. We developed a two-stage reconstruction procedure, and performed a total sacrectomy in 1982. This may be one of the earliest experiences of total sacrectomy in Japan. This case is described in Case 17 in Chap. 10, by A. Ogose and T. Morita, this volume and in detail in Chap. 6, by H.E. Takahashi, this volume.

Unique Reconstruction After a Type-II Resection of the Hip Joint Using the Ipsilateral Ankle Joint After Below-Knee Amputation

Reconstruction of the hip joint is the most difficult part of a type-II resection procedure (Enneking and Dunham 1978; Johnson 1978; O'Connor and Sim 1989; Steel 1978; Vena et al. 1999). The choices available include arthrodesis, a Sadle prosthesis, or a composite prosthesis. We developed an original procedure whereby the hip joint was reconstructed after an internal hemipelvectomy using a free osteoarticular vascularized graft consisting of the patient's ankle joint. Prior to the primary surgery, a below-knee (B/K) amputation of the ipsilateral limb was performed. The ankle joint from the amputated limb was then grafted to the resected hemipelvis, and functioned as the hip joint. After the surgery, the patient walked with a B/K prosthesis. This procedure is described in detail in Chap. 6, by H. Saito, this volume.

Reconstruction After a Type-III Resection Is not Necessary

There are few reports describing the reconstruction of the ischium and pubis (Enneking and Dunham 1978; O'Connor and Sim 1989). We carried out a multiinstitutional study of the clinical outcome of surgical treatment of ischiopubic bone tumors. The results indicated that reconstruction is not always necessary. This study is summarized in the following abstract of the Third Asia-Pacific Musculoskeletal Tumor Society Meeting (Hotta 2000).

Ischiopubic Bone Tumors

This multiinstitutional study was performed by the Japanese Musculoskeletal Oncology Group (JMOG) and involved 21 university hospitals and five cancer-center hospitals. The purpose of the study was to evaluate the clinical results of surgical treatment of primary ischiopubic bone tumors. The clinical outcome was assessed using a questionnaire. Seventy-one benign and 46 malignant bone tumors were registered. The mean follow-up period was 47.9 months. Eighty-four bone tumors occurred in the pubis, and 44 of these were benign. A solitary bone cyst was most frequently encountered (15 in number), followed by exostosis (10), and an aneurismal bone cyst (ABC, 9). Forty of the pubic bone tumors were malignant, with chondrosarcoma occurring most frequently (16), followed by osteosarcoma (OS, 11) and Ewing's sarcoma (ES, 7). Among the 27 benign ischial bone tumors, giant cell tumor (6) and eosinophilic granuloma (5) were the most common, followed by ABC (4) and fibrous dysplasia (4). Only six malignant ischial bone tumors were registered, with ES occurring most frequently. The prognosis of chondrosarcoma cases was excellent, with an 88% survival rate. However, the outcomes of the OS and ES cases were poor, with survival rates of 46% and 30%, respectively. Complications were encountered in 15% of all cases. Infection (7%) was the most frequent complication, followed by massive bleeding (2%). Only 4 out of the 36 patients with pubic resection without reconstruction experienced complaints such as pain with motion of the hip joint, herniation of a pelvic organ, pain in the sacroiliac joint, or edema in the limb.

It was concluded that the reconstruction of the pubis was not necessary except in particular cases. Surgery for OS and ES of the ischiopubic region remains a challenge.

Sacrificed Roots and Vesicorectal Disturbance

If one side of the S2 nerve root is intact, it is generally accepted that almost all vesicorectal function can be preserved. However, we treated a particular case of sacral chordoma arising in S3. The patient was an elderly man. A sacral amputation between the S1 and S2 levels was performed. By direct vision, both S2 roots were seen to be intact during surgery. After surgery, however, the patient lost the ability to urinate voluntarily. He also complained of severe constipation. We have also treated three similar cases. The innervation mechanism for vesicorectal function has not been clarified in the literature. Our experience leads us to doubt the current thinking on vesicorectal nerve control. Although we feel confident that the S3 root is necessary to maintain total vesicorectal function, we have very little experience to support this. It is important that the interaction of pelvic surgery and vesicorectal function be elucidated (see Case 9 in Chap. 10, by T. Hotta, this volume).

Quality of Life of Hemipelvectomy Patients

Is the quality of life of patients who have had a hemipelvectomy really poor? Reconstruction after the resection of a pelvic tumor is very difficult because of the possibility of infection or of the mechanical failure of the internal fixation device or prosthesis, or the effects of prolonged immobilization and inactivity. In addition, the cosmetic appearance of a hemipelvectomy is generally unacceptable. However, we know of several patients who have gone on to experience a very happy and fulfilled life. We must always consider a hemipelvectomy as a possible choice for pelvic surgery.

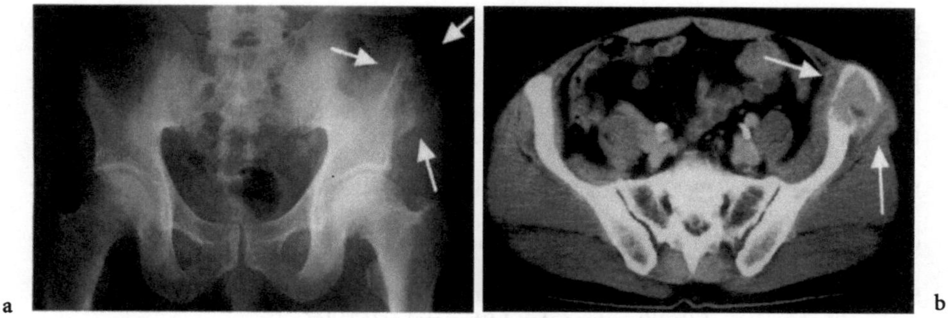

Fig. 1a,b. The case of a 66-year-old man with left renal cancer and pelvic bone metastasis. **a** X-ray film showing the osteolytic bone lesion with a thin cortical shell in the left ilium (*arrows*). Aspiration cytology revealed the features of a renal cell carcinoma. **b** CAT scan showing a thinned swollen cortex with low-density contents (*arrows*)

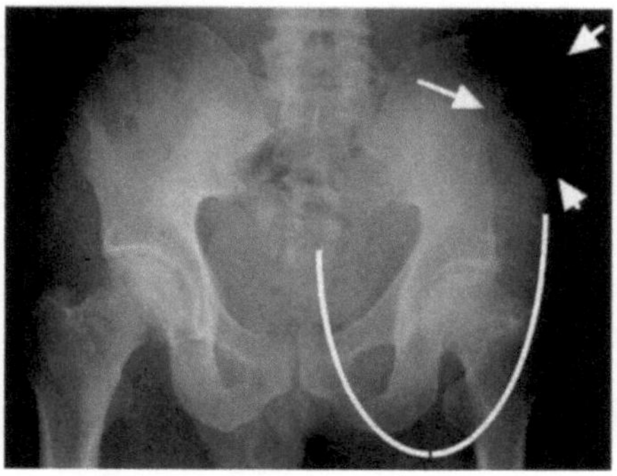

Fig. 2. No reconstruction was performed in this case (*arrows*). Five years after surgery, X-ray film shows neither local recurrence nor pelvic deformity. Massive bowel herniation occurs like the white U-shaped line when the patient stands up

Herniation of a Pelvic Organ

We have treated only one patient who experienced herniation of the bowel after resection of the ilium due to metastasis of a renal cell carcinoma. No reconstruction was attempted in this case (Figs. 1, 2). Massive herniation of the bowel can be observed in the standing position. No serious problems have occurred, although the patient does not feel well and is not satisfied with the result. The outcome would have been better if a mesh graft had been used to reconstruct the lower abdominal muscles and fascia.

References

Bergh PA, Bonamo J, Breen JL (1988) Pregnancy after hemipelvectomy: a case report and review of the literature. Int J Gynaecol Obstet 27:277–283

Enneking WF, Dunham WK (1978) Resection and reconstruction for primary neoplasms involving the innominate bone. J Bone Joint Surg Am 60:731–746

Holzaepfel JH (1973) Pregnancy and delivery post radical hemipelvectomy. Obstet Gynecol 42:455–458

Hotta T (2000) Ischiopubic bone tumors. Proceedigs of the 3rd Meeting of the Asia Pacific Musculoskeletal Tumor Society, Hong Kong, p 86

Johnson JT (1978) Reconstruction of the pelvic ring following tumor resection. J Bone Joint Surg Am 60:747–751

Nuss RC, Lee JH Jr (1967) Pregnancy following hemipelvectomy. Report of a case. Obstet Gynecol 29:789–791

O'Connor MI, Sim FH (1989) Salvage of the limb in the treatment of malignant pelvic tumors. J Bone Joint Surg Am 71:481–494

Snyder DJ, Thomas RL (1989) Pregnancy complicated by hemipelvectomy: case presentations and review of the literature. Am J Perinatol 6:363–366

Stavrakas PA, Sanders GT (1983) Sling support during pregnancy after hemipelvectomy: case report. Arch Phys Med Rehabil 64:331–333

Steel HH (1978) Partial or complete resection of the hemipelvis. An alternative to hindquarter amputation for periacetabular chondrosarcoma of the pelvis. J Bone Joint Surg Am 60:719–730

Vena VE, Hsu J, Rosier RN, O'Keefe RJ (1999) Pelvic reconstruction for severe periacetabular metastatic disease. Clin Orthop 362:171–180

Chapter 8
Complications

Complications and Sequelae

Takeshi Tojo

Summary. Pelvic tumor surgery has a high complication rate. Careful preoperative planning and team work with general, vascular, plastic, and urology surgeons are needed to control the complications.

Key words. Bleeding, Nerve damage, Infection

General Considerations

Complications at the Time of Surgery

The most frequent and serious intraoperative complication that occurs during pelvic surgery is massive bleeding. It is not uncommon that over 5000 ml of blood are lost during surgery for the removal of a large intrapelvic tumor. Careful planning with the anesthesiologist for blood transfusion is extremely important. When perioperative blood loss of more than 5000 ml is expected, a platelet transfusion should be prepared. Graft versus host disease, viral infection, or renal failure may develop after a large blood transfusion. Preoperative embolization is effective for highly vascular tumors such as a giant cell tumor or metastatic renal cell cancer.

Arterial bleeding is usually controlled by a ligation or suture technique. However, venous bleeding is difficult to control. When the sacrum is resected, Hata et al. (1998) recommended that the internal iliac veins should not be ligated in order to prevent venous congestion.

In several of our patients, the abdominal aorta was temporally pinched by an aortic clamp to control massive bleeding. This technique is extremely effective for uncontrollable bleeding, as described in Case 7 in Chap. 10, by Y.Z. Inoue, this volume.

Both local thrombosis and pulmonary thrombosis may develop with pelvic surgery. Fortunately, we have had no cases of pulmonary embolism at the time of surgery.

Postoperative Complications

Skin necrosis sometimes occurs after pelvic tumor surgery. The etiology of skin necrosis is multifocal. Contributing factors include the amount of soft tissue resection, the necessity of ligation of the feeding vessels, the shape of the skin flap, deep infection, postoperative hematoma, nutrition, anemia, and the location of the skin necrosis on the body. Care must be exercised so that only essential flaps are created, with a minimum of tension on the skin and soft tissue.

Infection often complicates the postoperative course in pelvic tumor surgery. Capanna et al. (1987) reported the incidence of postoperative infection to be 21%. Contributing factors include the amount of postoperative dead space, the duration of surgery, the development of skin necrosis, and postoperative chemotherapy. If infection is encountered, the treatment includes aggressive débridement and intravenous antibiotics. Ozaki et al. (1996) recommended filling the cavity with a bag of gentamycin beads in order to prevent postoperative infection in patients with a large sacral chordoma. It is sometimes advisable to obtain the assistance of a plastic surgeon for wound closure.

A bladder-skin fistula or bowel-skin fistula may develop after pelvic surgery. Careful monitoring of fistula output, including volume and composition, is important for subsequent management. Many low-output fistulas will heal spontaneously. High-output fistulas may require operative intervention, including laparotomy with bowel resection and anastomosis, interposed omentum, muscle flap interposition, or laparoscopic management (Chamberlain et al. 1998; Conlon and Boland 1997; Inmon and Bledsoe 1975).

Complications with Resection of the Sacrum

Nerve Damage

Resection of the sacral nerve roots is usually required in the treatment of a malignant sacral tumor. Subsequent bladder and rectal dysfunction after surgery are major complications. The extent of these problems depends upon the number and level of the nerve roots preserved. Even after a total sacrectomy with resection of both S1 nerve roots, patients can walk without a cane if adequate reconstruction is obtained between the lumbar spine and the pelvic ring. If the S2 nerve roots are sacrificed bilaterally, normal urogenic and rectal functions are lost. When both S2 nerve roots can be preserved, approximately half of all patients can regain at least partial bladder and bowel control. In patients with total unilateral loss of the sacral nerves, no significant anorectal or urinary impairment occurs (Carville 1995; Gunterberg et al. 1975, 1976).

Complications Involving Major Vessels

Thrombosis is a rare but often fatal complication. We have had one case of thrombosis in the left external iliac artery after a right hemipelvectomy. The exact cause was unknown. The patient underwent a thrombectomy, but circulation was still poor. Additional artificial vascular grafting was performed.

Postoperative bleeding from major vessels is also a potentially fatal complication. We have had one case where the external iliac artery was ruptured due to a postoperative infection, as described in Case 2 in Chap. 10, by H.E. Takahashi and T. Tojo, this volume.

Visceral Complications and Postoperative Causalgia

Urinary bladder or bowel damage is not uncommon, and requires intervention by a general surgeon and/or urologist. Causalgia may develop after resection of the upper sacral nerve roots. The pain is usually controllable with nonsteroidal antiinflammatory drugs (Fujimura et al. 1994).

Complications with Resection of the Ilium

Damage to the ureter may result from resection of the ilium. To prevent damage to the ureter in cases where it is surrounded by a large tumor, a urologist is often asked to place an intraureteral catheter before surgery in order to help in the location of the ureter. In a case of chordoma of the sacrum, oozing of urine from the scar tissue surrounding the ureter was noticed during disection. A J-shaped ureter catheter (double pigtail ureter catheter) was inserted before surgery. The catheter was kept in place after surgery, and eventually removed several weeks later. No further leakage of urine was noted. Hip dislocation and avascular necrosis of the femoral head may also occur with resection of the ilium.

Complications with Resection of the Pubis

The urinary bladder can be damaged when a pelvic tumor invades the pelvic cavity. Massive bleeding may develop if the corpus cavernosum of the penis is damaged.

Complications with Resection of the Ischium

After a hemipelvectomy with total resection of the ischium, patients often experience instability when sitting. When the ischium can be partially preserved, the pelvic ring can be reconstructed using the fibula from the resected limb in order to improve postoperative stability when sitting (Fig. 1) (Ogose et al. 1993).

a,b

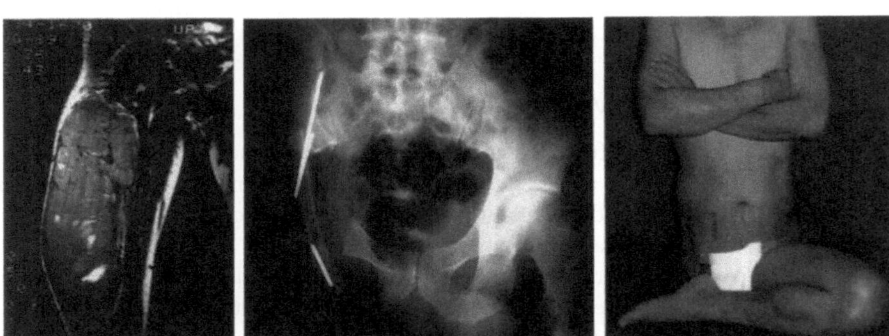

c

FIG. 1. **a** Magnetic resonance image showing a recurrent hemangiopericytoma of the proximal thigh. **b** Plain radiograph showing reconstruction of the pelvic ring using a free fibula graft after modified hemipelvectomy. **c** Postoperative photograph showing the patient in a stable sitting position

References

Capanna R, van Horn JR, Guernelli N, Briccoli A, Ruggieri P, Biagini R, Bettellini G, Campanacci M (1987) Complications of pelvic resections. Arch Orthop Trauma Surg 106:71–77

Carville K (1995) Caring for cancerous wounds in the community. J Wound Care 4:66–68

Chamberlain RS, Kaufman HL, Danforth DN (1998) Enterocutaneous fistula in cancer patients: etiology, management, outcome, and impact on further treatment. Am Surg 64:1204–1211

Conlon KC, Boland PJ (1997) Laparoscopically assisted radical sacrococcygectomy. A new operative approach to large sacrococcygeal chordomas. Surg Endosc 11:1118–1122

Fujimura Y, Maruiwa H, Takahata T, Toyama Y (1994) Neurological evaluation after radical resection of sacral neoplasms. Paraplegia 32:396–406

Gunterberg B, Norlen L, Stener B, Sundin T (1975) Neurourologic evaluation after resection of the sacrum. Invest Urol 13:183–188

Gunterberg B, Kewenter J, Petersen I, Stener B (1976) Anorectal function after major resections of the sacrum with bilateral or unilateral sacrifice of sacral nerves. Br J Surg 63:546–554

Hata M, Kawahara N, Tomita K (1998) Influence of ligation of the internal iliac veins on the venous plexuses around the sacrum. J Orthop Sci 3:264–271

Inmon WB, Bledsoe JW (1975) Surgical repair of genital prolapse after hemipelvectomy. Am J Obstet Gynecol 123:766–769

Ogose A, Saito H, Inoue YZ, Hotta T, Otsuka H, Yamamura S, Takahashi HE (1993) Hemipelvectomy for primary and metastatic malignant tumors (in Japanese). Rinsho Seikei Geka (Clinical Orthopaedic Surgery) 28:1097–1103

Ozaki T, Hillmann A, Bettin D, Wuisman P, Winkelmann W (1996) High complication rates with pelvic allografts. Experience of 22 sarcoma resections. Acta Orthop Scand 67: 333–338

Chapter 9
Outcomes

Oncological and Functional Outcomes, Vesicorectal Dysfunction, and Complications

Tetsuo Hotta

Summary. Some oncological and functional outcomes of surgical treatment of pelvic tumors are described. Seventy-four bone tumors and 16 soft tissue tumors were included in this study. Fifty-two bone tumors were malignant and 22 were benign. Ten soft tissue tumors were malignant and six were benign. The local cure rate was poor in type II (acetabular) and type IV (sacral) bone tumors. The local recurrence rate for type II and type IV bone tumor was 40.0% and 47.1%, respectively. The cumulative 5-year survival rate for type-II bone tumors was the worst at only 40%. Limb function was also poor in type-II bone tumors. Vesicorectal dysfunction was also observed when both S2 nerve roots were spared.

Key words. Oncological outcome, Functional outcome, Vesicorectal dysfunction, Sacral amputation, Infection

Introduction

This chapter summarizes the oncological and functional outcomes of our surgical treatment of pelvic tumors from 1965 to 2000, inclusive. The outcomes were also evaluated according to histological diagnoses. The bone tumors were divided into four types based on their location: type I, ilium; type II, acetabulum; type III, ischiopubic; type IV, sacrum. Large tumors, which occupied portions of the acetabulum and ilium, or the acetabulum and ischiopubic bone, or the acetabulum, ilium, and ischiopubic bone, were included as type-II tumors. Soft tissue tumors were categorized as occurring either inside or outside the pelvis, and were classified as being located either in the buttock, the intrapelvic region, or the inguinal region.

The oncological outcomes of malignant tumors and giant cell tumors were evaluated by the local recurrence rate, and the cumulative survival rate as determined by the method of Kaplan–Meier (Kaplan and Meier 1958). The functional outcome was assessed by Enneking's method (Enneking et al. 1993) for the evaluation of spared limb function. Vesicorectal dysfunction in patients with type-IV tumors was evaluated by our own method, which was based on the assignment of one of four grades (0–3 points). Three points represent normal function, two points indicate a slight disturbance of vesicorectal function with occasional incontinence or constipation, one point indicates completely uncontrolled vesicorectal function, and a zero score indicates urinary diversion or colostomy.

The cases of surgically treated pelvic bone tumors are summarized in Tables 1–5. Seventy-four bone tumors and 16 soft tissue tumors were included. Twenty-seven of the bone tumors were type I, 12 were type II, 14 were type III, and 21 were type IV. Fifty-two of the bone tumors were malignant and 22 were benign. Giant cell tumors (GCTs) were included with malignant bone tumors in this study. Ten of the soft tissue tumors were malignant and six were benign. Chondrosarcoma was the most frequently encountered malignant bone tumor, followed by osteosarcoma and Ewing's sarcoma. Cancer metastasis was also operated on in eight cases. Renal cell carcinoma was the most frequently encountered cancer among the metastasis cases operated on. Aneurysmal bone cyst was the most common benign bone tumor, followed by a solitary bone cyst and then exostosis.

TABLE 1. Summary of 27 cases with type-I bone tumors

Average age	Male : female	Histological diagnosis	Number of cases	Malignant		Benign
				LS	Hemipelvectomy	
30.8	15 : 12			12	8	7
	Malignant	Chondrosarcoma	8			
		Ewing's sarcoma	2			
		MFH	1			
		Malignant GCT	1			
		Fibrosarcoma	1			
		Malignant lymphoma	1			
		Cancer metastasis	5			
		GCT	1			
	Benign	Eosinophilic granuloma	3			
		ABC	2			
		SBC	2			

LS, limb salvage; MFH, malignant fibrous histiocytoma; GCT, giant cell tumor of bone; ABC, aneurysmal bone cyst; SBC, solitary bone cyst

TABLE 2. Summary of 12 cases with type-II bone tumors

Average age	Male : female	Histological diagnosis	Number of cases	Malignant		Benign
				LS	Hemipelvectomy	
50.8	8 : 4			8	2	2
	Malignant	Chondrosarcoma	4			
		Osteosarcoma	2			
		Ewing's sarcoma	1			
		Cancer metastasis	2			
		GCT	1			
	Benign	Fibromyxoma	1			
		BFH	1			

BFH, benign fibrous histiocytoma

TABLE 3. Summary of 14 cases with type-III bone tumors

Average age	Male:female	Histological diagnosis	Number of cases	Malignant		Benign
				LS	Hemipelvectomy	
31.8	8:6			4	1	9
	Malignant	Chondrosarcoma	3			
		Osteosarcoma	2			
	Benign	Exostosis	3			
		ABC	3			
		SBC	2			
		Hemangioma	1			

TABLE 4. Summary of 21 cases with type-IV bone tumors

Average age	Male:female	Histological diagnosis	Number of cases	Malignant		Benign
				LS	Hemipelvectomy	
50.3	13:8			16	1	4
	Malignant	Chordoma	8			
		Chondrosarcoma	3			
		Malignant schwannoma	1			
		Cancer metastasis	1			
		GCT	4			
	Benign	Schwannoma	4			

TABLE 5. Summary of 16 cases with soft tissue tumors

Average age	Male:female	Histological diagnosis	Number of cases	Malignant		Benign
				LS	Hemipelvectomy	
50.6	4:12			10	0	6
	Malignant	Liposarcoma	4			
		Malignant schwannoma	2			
		Desmoid	3			
		Synovial sarcoma	1			
	Benign	Schwannoma	4			
		Myxoma	1			
		Chronic expanding hematoma	1			

Oncological Outcome

Local Recurrence Rate

In benign bone tumors, only one local recurrence of hemangioma was observed. The overall recurrence rate was 32.5% for malignant bone tumors and 50.0% for malignant soft tissue tumors. Individual recurrence rates for types I, II, III, and IV bone tumors were 20.0%, 40.0%, 20.0%, and 47.1%, respectively. The local recurrence rates of types II and IV were high because the resection procedure was anatomically difficult in type-II bone tumors, and the tumors were usually very large in type-IV bone tumors. In spite of a wide resection, many cases of type-IV sacral bone tumors exhibited local recurrence.

The local recurrence rate for chondrosarcoma was significantly lower than that with other high-grade tumors such as osteosarcoma or Ewing's sarcoma. There was no recurrence in the one case of malignant fibrous histiocytoma (MFH) of the ilium. The MFH in this case was of the inflammatory type, and the patient was treated with chemotherapy and preoperative radiation therapy. A hemipelvectomy was performed, and the resected specimen exhibited complete necrosis. This was thought to be a rare case.

Cumulative Survival Rate (Primary Malignant Tumor and GCT)

Cases of benign tumors and metastatic tumors were excluded from this analysis. The survival rates are shown in Figs. 1 and 2. The overall 5-year survival rates for patients with malignant bone tumors and soft tissue tumors were 57.7% and 90%, respectively. Individual survival rates for patients with types I, II, III, and IV tumors were 64.6%, 40.0%, 100%, and 58.3%, respectively. The survival rate for patients with type-II bone tumors was much worse.

The survival rate for patients with chondrosarcoma was significantly higher than that for patients with other tumors. There were no specific trends in the survival rates of patients with soft tissue sarcomas.

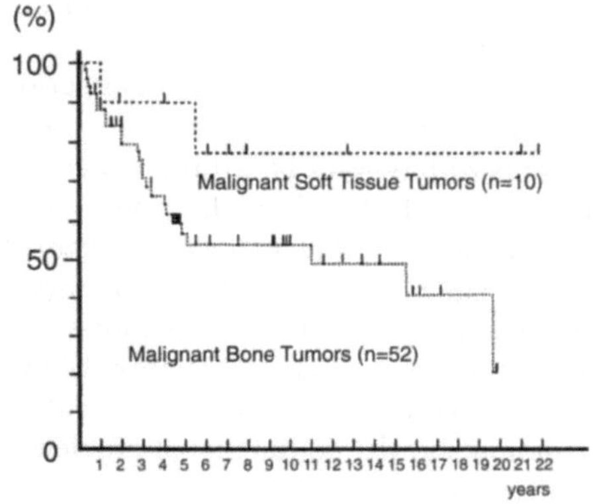

FIG. 1. Kaplan–Meier survival curve for malignant bone and soft tissue tumors. The cumulative 5-year survival rate for all types of malignant bone tumors is calculated to be 57.7%. The survival rate for malignant soft tissue tumors is 90%, which is significantly better than that for malignant bone tumors

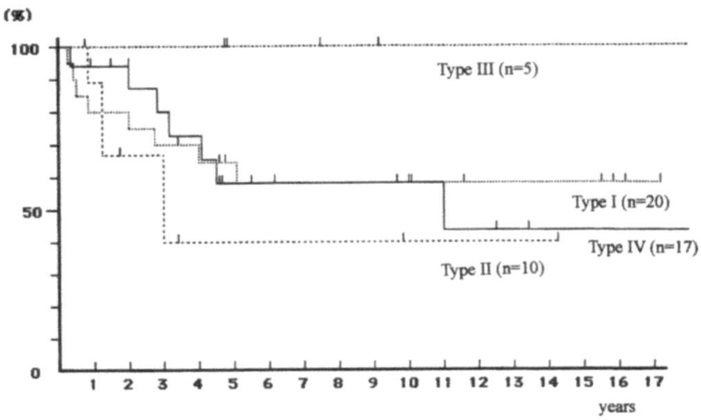

FIG. 2. Individual cumulative survival curve for types I, II, III, and IV malignant bone tumors. The cumulative 5-year survival rate for type-II tumors is the worst

Functional Outcome

Limb Function

Benign tumor cases and hemipelvectomy cases were excluded from the functional evaluation. Hemipelvectomy was performed in 12 of 52 malignant bone tumor cases. The rates of limb salvage of types I, II, III, and IV tumors were 60.0%, 80.0%, 80.0%, and 94.1%, respectively. In the early days of our use of pelvic surgery, hemipelvectomy was the only method. Therefore, many of our type-I cases might have been the candidates for limb salvage surgery today. Limb salvage procedures were perfomed in all malignant soft tissue tumor cases and in 40 malignant bone tumor cases, including cases with a GCT.

Enneking's evaluation system for limb function is shown in Table 6 (Enneking et al. 1993). The functions of patients with types I, II, III, IV and soft tissue tumors were 85.8%, 56.3%, 100%, 69.2%, and 86.0%, respectively. Our cases demonstrated that reconstruction of the hip joint is very difficult. We have only limited experience of such reconstruction, and these cases are summarized in Table 7. Limb function with total hip arthroplasty seems to be superior to that following arthrodesis according to our functional evaluation at a short-term follow up. The functional outcomes of patients with type-IV bone tumors were also worse owing to the sacrifice of the spinal nerve roots of S1 and/or L4,5. Some patients were suffering from pain, which originated in a nerve injury or in a structural problem of sacroiliac joint or lumboiliac fusion. The problem with type-I tumors was mainly based on the reconstruction of the iliosacral joint. However, the total function of patients with limb salvage after a type-I bone tumor was satisfactory. All four type-III cases showed excellent function. A bony reconstruction was carried out in three cases, and one case without reconstruction showed no functional problem. Bony reconstruction of the pubis may not be necessary.

TABLE 6. Enneking's system of functional evaluation

Points	Pain	Function	Emotional Acceptance	Supports	Walking	Gait
5	None	No restriction	Enthused	None	Unlimited	Normal
4	Intermediate	Intermediate	Intermediate	Intermediate	Intermediate	Intermediate
3	Modest	Recreational restriction	Satisfied	Brace	Limited	Minor, cosmetic
2	Intermediate	Intermediate	Intermediate	Intermediate	Intermediate	Intermediate
1	Moderate	Partial disability	Accepts	1 cane, 1 crutch	Inside only	Major cosmetic, minor HCAP
0	Severe	Total disability	Dislikes	2 canes, 2 crutches	Not independently	Major HCAP

HCAP, handicap

TABLE 7. Reconstruction of the hip joint after type-II resection

Age	Sex	Diagnosis	Reconstruction procedure	Limb function (%)	FU (months)	Outcome
26	M	GCT	Arthrodesis	73	174	CDF
55	M	Chondrosarcoma	Arthrodesis	53	121	CDF
30	F	Osteosarcoma	Osteoarticular Graft	30	15	DOD
67	M	Metastasis (RCC)	THA	60	36	DOD
62	F	Chondrosarcoma	THA	67	44	CDF
65	F	Chondrosarcoma	Constrained THA[a]	37	12	CDF
12	M	Ewing's sarcoma	Ankle graft[b]	30	15	DOD

FU, follow-up; THA, total hip arthroplasty; CDF, continuously disease-free; DOD, dead of disease

[a] The cup was placed in the sacrum

[b] The ipsilateral ankle joint was grafted as a free vascularized osteoarticular graft after below-knee amputation

Vesicorectal Dysfunction with Type-IV Tumors

We had seven cases with sacral amputation. Their vesicorectal dysfunction and amputation levels are summarized in Table 8. Palliative curettage cases, hemisacrectomy cases, and total sacrectomy cases were excluded. Whenever malignant lesions of the sacrum are resected, vesicorectal dysfunction will always occur. There does not seem to be a clear-cut relationship between the amputation level and vesicorectal dysfunction. As mentioned in Chap. 7, by T. Morita, the function of the S2 root is not clearly understood. Based on our results, the S3 root may play an essential role in the maintenance of normal vesicorectal function. We do not have enough cases with which to investigate the relationship between amputation level and sexual function.

TABLE 8. Amputation level of the sacrum and vesicorectal dysfunction

Age	Sex	Diagnosis	Amputation level	VRD	Limb function (%)	FU (months)	Outcome
58	M	Chordoma	S 2/3	2	63	49	DOD
67	F	Chordoma	S 2/3	2	87	54	DOD
51	M	Chordoma	S 1/2	0	100	150	AWD
41	M	GCT	S 1/2	2	100	111	CDF
40	M	Chordoma	S 2/3	2	100	55	CDF
78	M	Chordoma	S 2/3	2	100	24	CDF
69	M	Chordoma	S 2/3	1	100	18	CDF

VRD, vesicorectal dysfunction; AWD, alive with disease

Furthermore, since most of the patients in this study were elderly, one would expect there to be a decrease in sexual function as a natural consequence of the aging process.

Complications

No complications occurred in benign bone tumors. Complications were observed in 25.0% of patients with malignant bone tumors, and in 20.0% of all soft tissue tumors. Infection occurred in three of 52 cases with malignant bone tumors. Open treatment was needed in three cases with type-IV bone tumors owing to the large dead space. A complication-related death occurred in one case of sacral GCT. Two infections were observed in patients with malignant soft tissue tumors, and one case of massive bleeding was observed in a patient with a benign soft tissue tumor.

References

Enneking WF, Dunham W, Gebhardt MC, Malawar M, Pritchard DJ (1993) A system for the functional evaluation of reconstructive procedures after surgical treatment of tumors of the musculoskeletal system. Clin Orthop 286:214–246

Kaplan EL, Meier P (1958) Nonparametric estimation for incomplete observations. J Am Stat Assoc 53:457–481

Chapter 10
Case Presentations

Case 1: Resection of a Giant Cell Tumor of the Sacrum, and Unilateral Reconstruction of the Sacroiliac Joint in a 51-Year-Old Woman

HIDEAKI E. TAKAHASHI

Summary. A giant cell tumor of the sacrum, initially thought to be a herniated lumbar disc, was resected, including the sacroiliac joint. Reconstruction of the osseous pelvic ring was performed using autogenous bone from the fibula and iliac crest.

Key words. Giant cell tumor, Sacroiliac joint, Fibula graft, Sacrectomy, Radiation therapy

Clinical History

The patient developed pain in the left buttock in 1981. She initially received surgical treatment for suspected herniation of a lumbar disc (Fig. 1). At the time of surgery, however, a bone tumor was detected. A biopsy revealed a giant cell tumor of the sacrum. The patient was referred to the Niigata University Hospital (Fig. 2). She began to experience urinary incontinence and pain with bowel movement soon after admission. Neurological examination revealed a sensory disturbance. Dysesthesia and hypesthesia of the lateral aspect of the left buttock, thigh, leg, and foot below the S1 level were detected. Hypesthesia of the right perianal region below the S4 level was also detected. The left ankle jerk was absent. Arteriography revealed the retention of contrast medium in the left side of the sacrum (Fig. 3).

Surgical Procedure

A subtotal sacrectomy was performed in August 1981, and included the left sacroiliac joint. Through a divergent U-shaped skin incision, a left pararectal incision was made below the level of the umbilicus, transecting the rectus abdominus just 1 cm above the pubic symphysis (Fig. 4). Extraperitoneal dissection was performed, and the left internal iliac artery and vein were doubly ligated and transected. The anterior pseudocapsule of the tumor was then exposed, followed by dissection of the left sacroiliac joint laterally, the upper border of the left side of the sacrum superiorly, and the lower border of the sacrum inferiorly. The left L5 and S1 nerve roots were entrapped within the tumor, and were transected at the level of the sciatic notch. A right pararectal incision was then made, and the rectus abdominus was detached from the pubic symphysis, exposing the anterior surface of the right side of the sacrum. An osteotomy

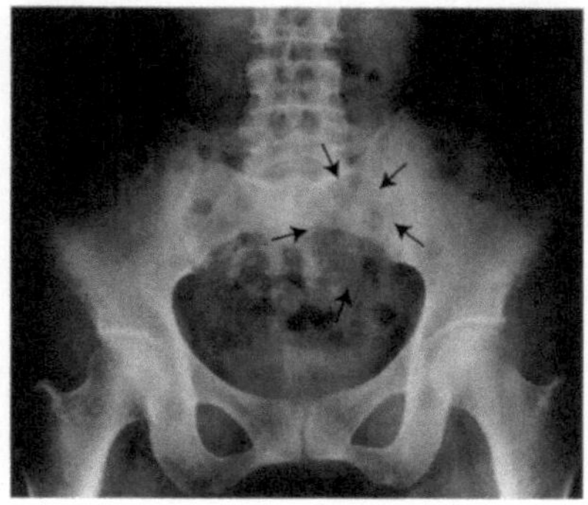

FIG. 1. Anteroposterior (AP) view of the pelvis showing an osteolytic tumor located in the left side of the sacrum (June 24, 1981)

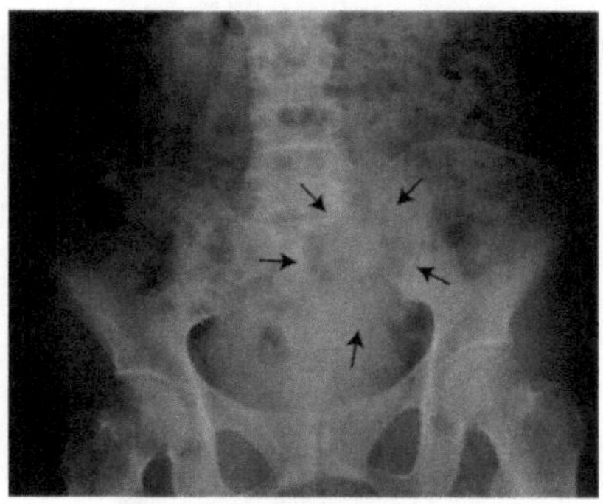

FIG. 2. AP view of the pelvis showing an osteolytic tumor in the left side of the sacrum (August 11, 1981)

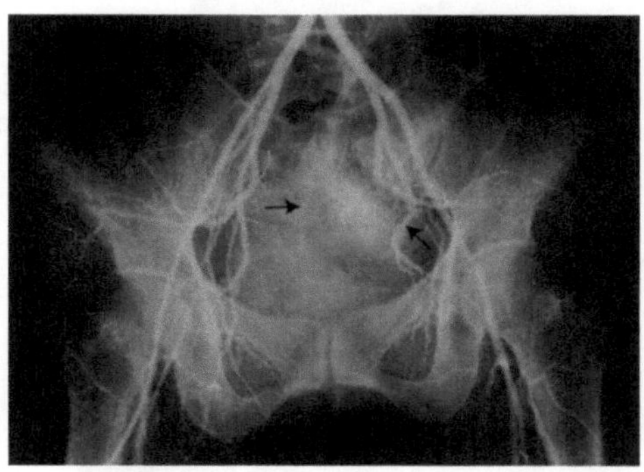

FIG. 3. AP view of arteriography revealing retention of the contrast medium in the left side of the sacrum (July 22, 1981)

of the sacrum was performed by connecting the neural foramina of the right S1, S2, and S3 vertebra, which were all preserved.

The patient was then changed from the supine position to the prone position. A posterior midline skin incision was made from L3 to the coccyx, and was extended to the left and laterally to the level of L4, and to the left and slightly inferiorly-laterally to the level of the coccyx. The left gluteus maximus was split, and the osteotomy line of the left ilium was exposed toward the left sciatic notch. The piriformis muscle, sacrotuberous ligament, and sacrospinous ligament were transected, and the inferior

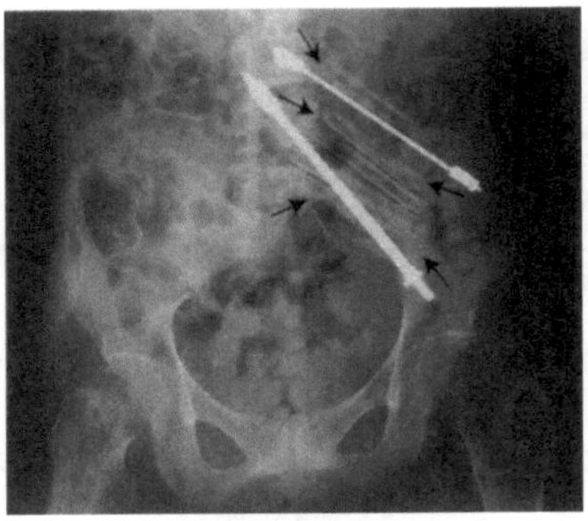

FIG. 4. Lumbosacroiliac joint reconstructed with an autogenous fibula and ilium after wide resection (July 8, 1982). The reconstruction was augmented with a distraction rod placed between L4 and the ilium, and a compression rod placed between L3 and the ilium

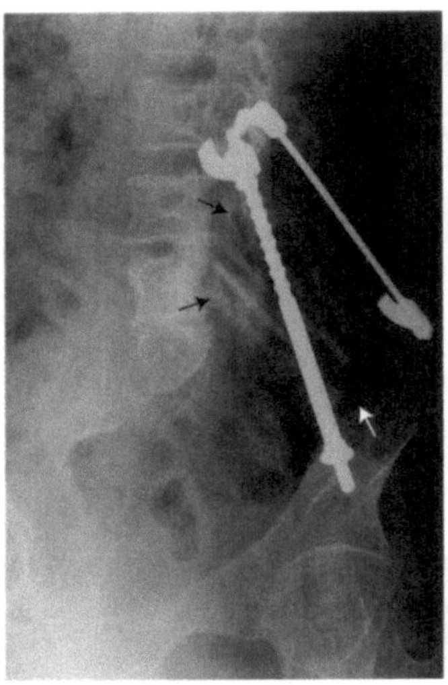

FIG. 5. Oblique view of the reconstructed lumbosacroiliac joint (November 15, 1982)

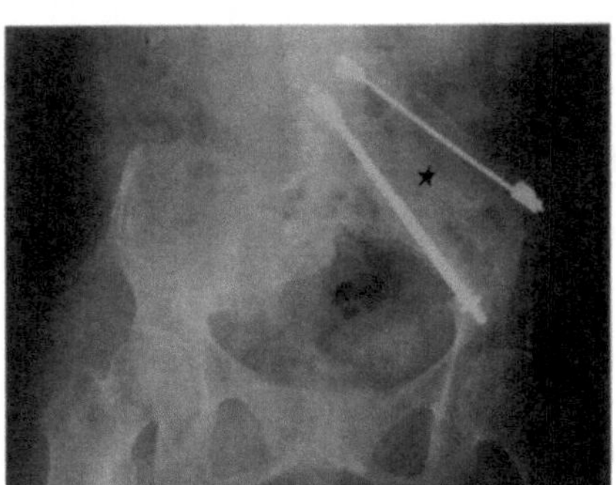

FIG. 6. Lumbosacroiliac joint reconstructed with autogenous bone from the fibula and ilium (January 10, 1991). The grafts were incorporated from bone remodeling, and the left femur was atrophied due to partial weight bearing. *, well homogenized grafted bone

gluteal artery and vein were ligated and transected. Laminectomies of L4, L5, the sacrum, and a portion of L3 were performed, and there revealed that the tumor occupied the left epidural space of L5 to S3. The left L5, S1, and S2 nerve roots were entrapped within the tumor, and were severed. The tumor tissue was scraped off the dura. All other sacral nerve roots were preserved intact. A portion of the anterior osteotomy line was visible. The osteotomy was then completed posteriorly, and the osteotomized bone mass, including the tumor, was removed. The large dead space was left unfilled. A secondary closure was performed 2 months later. After the skin incision healed, radiation therapy was administered with a total dose of 5600 rad.

Reconstructive surgery was performed by placing a bone bridge between the left ilium and the residual sacrum using autogenous bone from the fibula and ilium. These grafts were transfixed by providing a compressive force with a Harrington compression rod, and a distraction force with a threaded wire (Fig. 5).

Nine years after surgery, the patient could walk with a pair of crutches (Fig. 6). Nineteen years after surgery, she was still living, had no recurrence of the tumor, and still walked with a pair of crutches.

Case 2: Treatment of a Giant Cell Tumor of the Sacrum in a 27-Year-Old Man, Using Four Struts at the Lumbosacral Level to Support the Trunk

HIDEAKI E. TAKAHASHI

Summary. A giant cell tumor of the sacrum, occupying nearly the entire pelvic cavity, was detected. The patient developed constipation, and experienced a sensation that his trunk was sinking into his pelvis. Partial resection of the tumor and radiation therapy were carried out. Subsequently, the patient could walk and returned to work. A calcified residual tumor began to grow a year and a half later. Further resection was complicated by local infection and bleeding from the external iliac artery.

Key words. Four struts, Giant cell tumor, Fibula graft, Radiation therapy, Constipation

Clinical History

The patient developed pain in the coccygeal region in February 1981. He was initially thought to have had a discogenic lesion, and was treated conservatively. However, he developed constipation 7 months later. Myelography revealed a radiolucent lesion in the sacrum. A biopsy was obtained, and the lesion was diagnosed as a giant cell tumor. The patient was referred to Niigata University Hospital 8 months after the onset of symptoms.

On admission, the patient complained of pain in the lower back and difficulty with walking because of a sensation that his trunk was sinking into his pelvis. It was found that his sacrum had almost been replaced by an osteolytic tumor that occupied nearly the entire pelvic cavity (Figs. 1, 2). The treatment plan was as follows: surgical placement of four struts to support the trunk, radiotherapy to control the growth of the tumor, and reduction of the tumor mass.

Surgical Procedure

In November 1981, partial resection of the tumor was performed, and two Harrington distraction rods from L3 laminae to a sacral bar were placed between the bilateral ilia to act as two posterior struts. The patient was then treated with a total of 5940 rad of radiation. In June 1982, anterior struts using bilateral fibulae were grafted between the third lumbar spine and the ilium, close to the sacroiliac joint line. After gait training, the patient could walk again without external support, and no longer

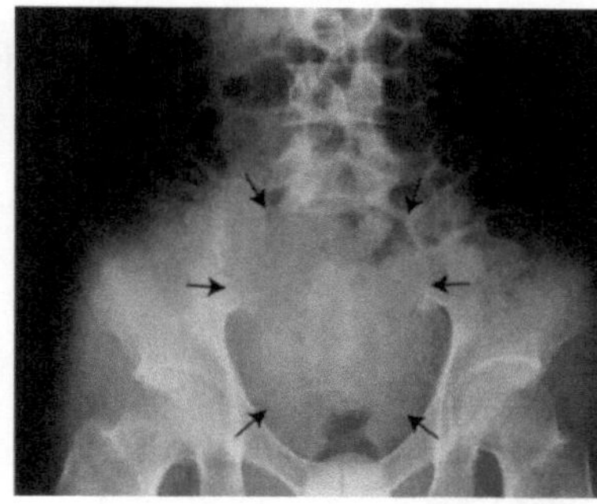

FIG. 1. Anteroposterior (AP) view of the pelvis revealing an osteolytic tumor in the sacrum (October 29, 1981). The sacrum had almost entirely been replaced by the tumor tissue

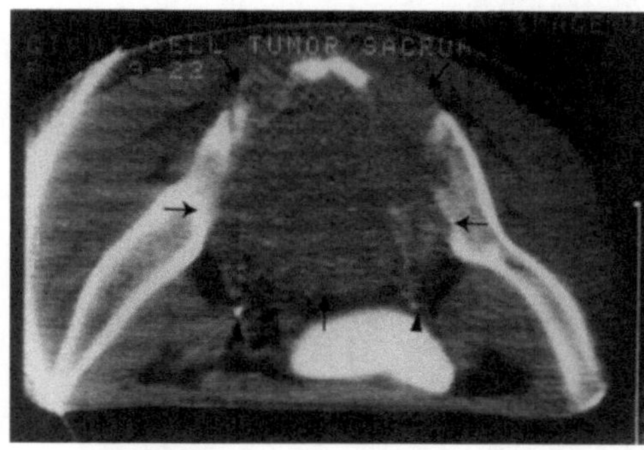

FIG. 2. Computed tomography (CT) scan showing that the sacral tumor protruded extraosseously into the pelvic cavity, and expanded submuscularly (October 24, 1981). ▲, ureter

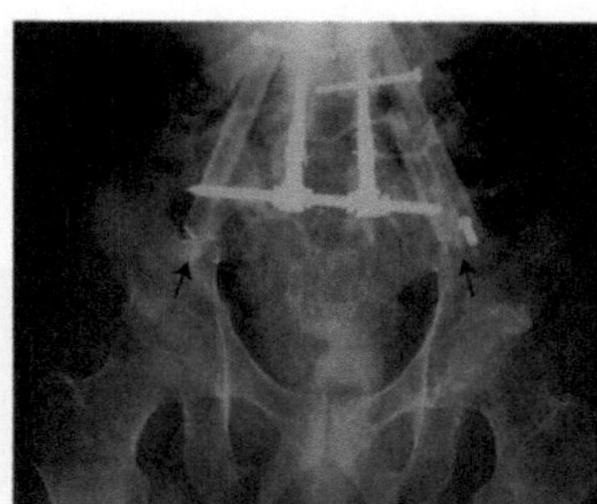

FIG. 3. AP view of the lumbosacroiliac region reconstructed with four struts consisting of bilateral anterior fibular grafts and bilateral posterior Harrington distraction rods (March 24, 1983)

had the sinking sensation. In 1983, he was ambulatory and returned to his regular work. The radiolucent tumor had calcified and decreased in size (Figs. 3–5). In March 1984, a computerized tomography scan showed regrowth of the tumor (Fig. 6). In September 1984, wide resection of the tumor and sacrum was performed, together with a partial resection of an ureterocutaneous fistula and the right ureter, which was surrounded by the tumor. Cubes of hydroxyapatite were implanted in the defect.

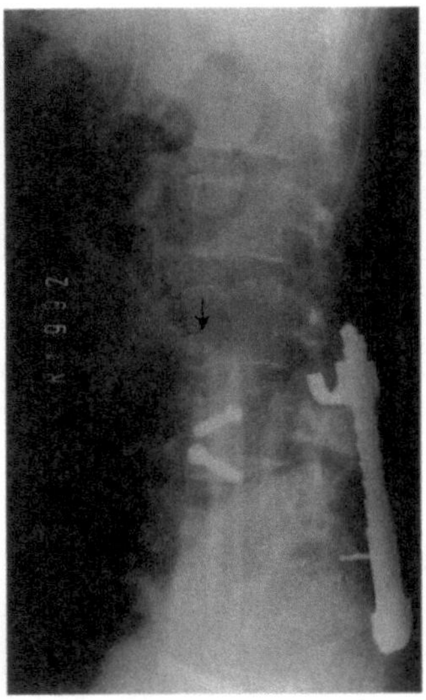

Fig. 4. AP view of the reconstructed lumbosacroiliac region with the four struts (March 24, 1983)

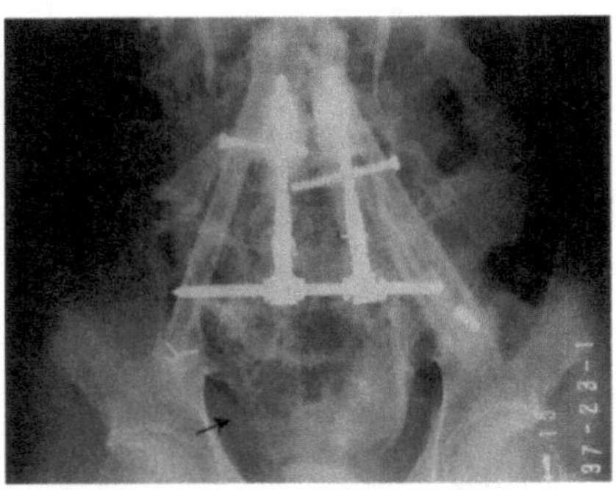

Fig. 5. AP view of the reconstructed lumbosacroiliac region with the four struts (July 27, 1983)

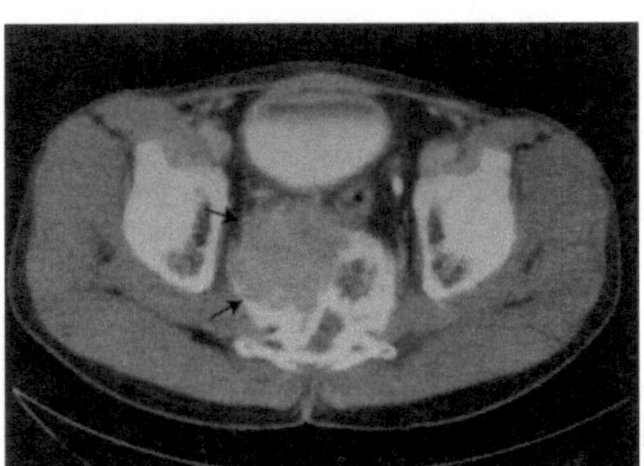

Fig. 6. CT scan of the sacral tumor, which was partially calcified and had expanded into the pelvic cavity (August 1, 1984)

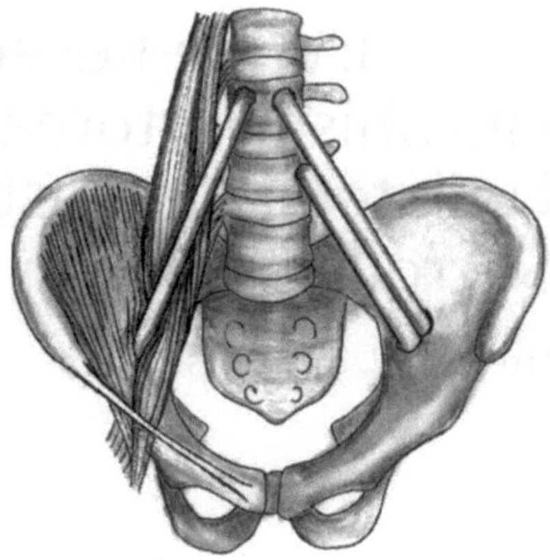

FIG. 7. Schematic AP view of the lumbosacroiliac region reconstructed as bilateral anterior struts with fibular grafts connecting the anterior portion of the vertebral body of L3 and the pelvis (March 24, 1983)

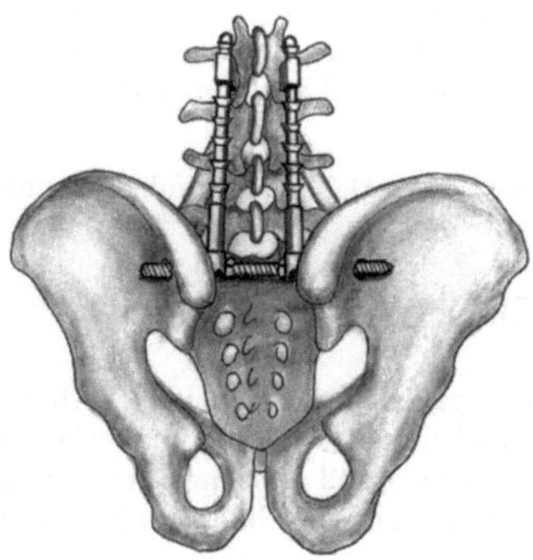

FIG. 8. Schematic posteroanterior view of the lumbosacroiliac region reconstructed as bilateral posterior struts with Harrington distraction rods connecting lamina of L3 and a sacral bar, inserted between the bilateral ilia (March 24, 1983)

Postoperative Course

Approximately 1 month after resection of the tumor, massive bleeding occurred from the right external iliac artery. Bleeding recurred 1 week later. The patient's postoperative course was also complicated by local infection and severe hepatic and renal failure, which necessitated temporary hemodialysis. The patient died on January 24, 1985.

Case 3: Wide Resection of a Malignant Fibrohistiocytoma of the Ilium and Unilateral Reconstruction of the Sacroiliac Joint in a 28-Year-Old Man

Hideaki E. Takahashi

Summary. A malignant fibrohistiocytoma of the ilium, initially diagnosed as a giant cell bone tumor, was treated with curettage and homogenous bone grafting. A radiolucent bone tumor was detected 14 years after this first operative procedure. An open biopsy revealed a malignant fibrohistiocytoma of the same lesions. Resection of the tumor and osseous reconstruction of the sacroiliac joint were performed.

Key words. Malignant fibrohistiocytoma, Sacroiliac joint, Fibula graft, Ilium

Clinical History

The patient developed pain in the left hip in 1962. Eight months later, he was found to have an osteolytic lesion in the left ilium (Fig. 1). An open biopsy was performed, and a diagnosis of giant cell tumor was made. The lesion was curetted, and homogenous bone grafting was performed. The postoperative course was uneventful. At the follow-up examination in 1966, no sign of any recurrence of the tumor was recorded. In 1972, the region of the previous surgery showed an osteosclerotic and partially osteolytic lesion (Figs. 2 and 3). The patient was examined twice during the following year, but it was felt that he did not have a definitive recurrence of the tumor.

In 1986, the patient developed pain in the left hip. Osteolytic lesions were detected in the region of the previous operation in the left ilium, and in the left side of the sacrum, across from the left sacroiliac joint (Figs. 4 and 5). A malignant fibrohistiocytoma was diagnosed after an open biopsy.

Surgical Procedure

In February 1986, a wide resection of the tumor was performed with the patient in the right lateral position. The patient was placed in a semisupine position for anterior dissection of the tumor, which was located in the medial third of the ilium and in the left side of the sacrum. For posterior dissection of the left ilium and sacrum, the patient was slightly rotated to the semiprone position, keeping the right lateral

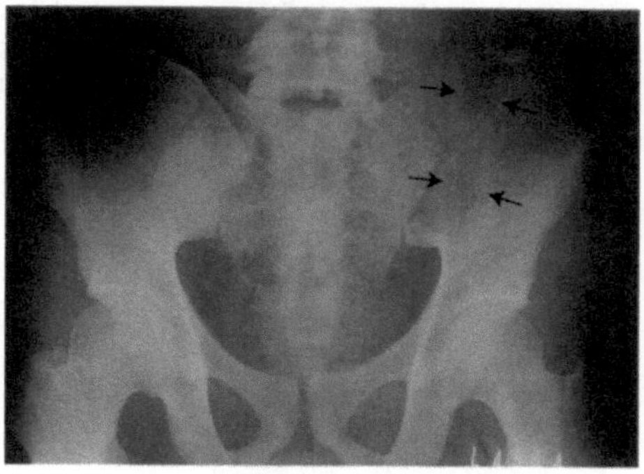

FIG. 1. Anteroposterior (AP) view of the osteolytic tumor in the left ilium (June 22, 1963)

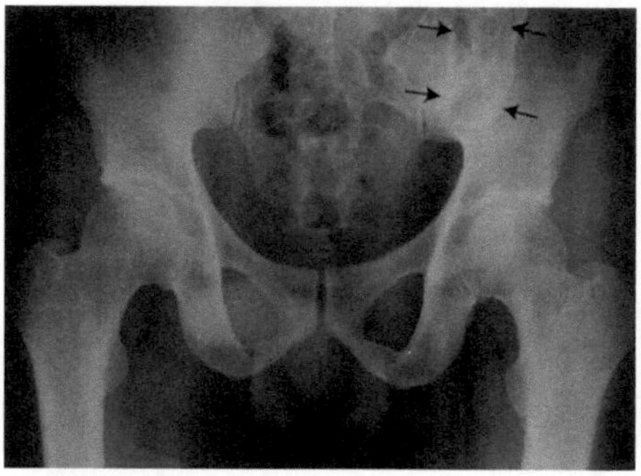

FIG. 2. AP view of the osteosclerotic lesion in the left ilium, which had previously been curetted and had received a homogenous bone graft (December 20, 1972)

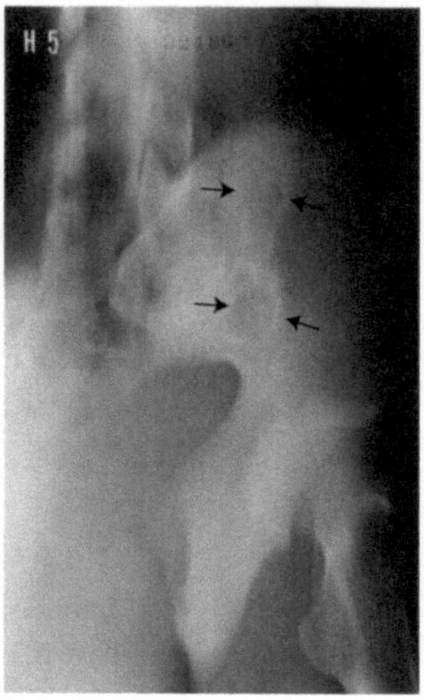

FIG. 3. Oblique view of the osteosclerotic lesion in the left ilium (February 16, 1973)

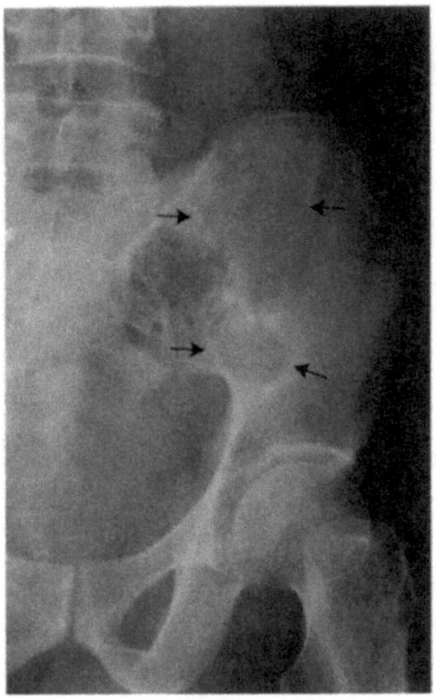

Fig. 4. AP view of the osteolytic tumor in the left ilium and sacrum, which was diagnosed as a malignant fibrohistiocytoma (January 13, 1986)

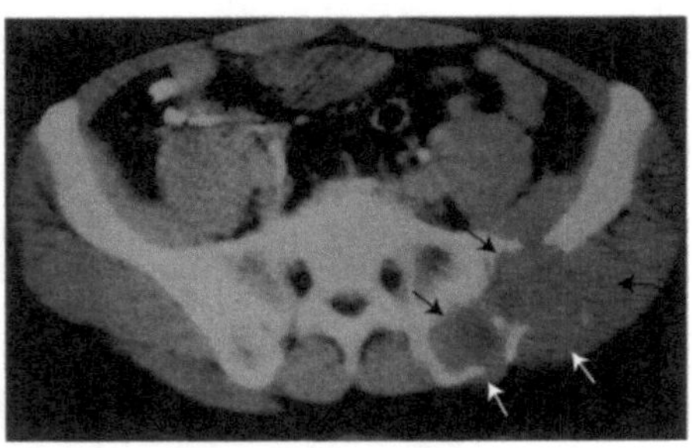

Fig. 5. A computed tomography scan showing an osteolytic tumor in the left ilium and sacrum, which had expanded extraosseously under the gluteus maximus (January 1986)

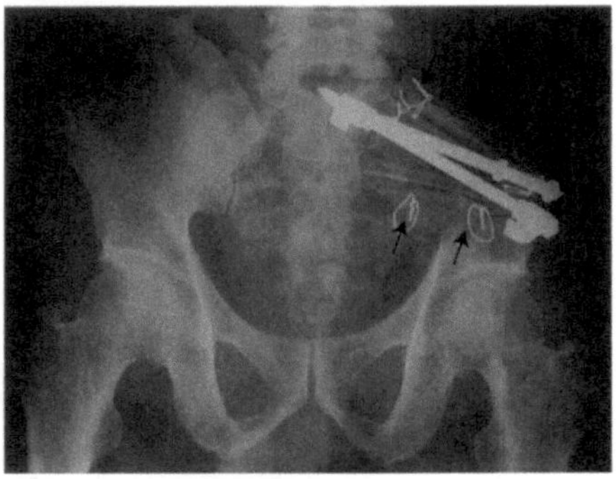

Fig. 6. AP view of the defect in the left sacroiliac joint, which had been reconstructed with a split autogenous fibular bone graft. The graft was augmented with a Harrington distraction rod, which generated a compressive force on the reconstruction, and a threaded sacral bar, which generated a tensile force (April 17, 1986)

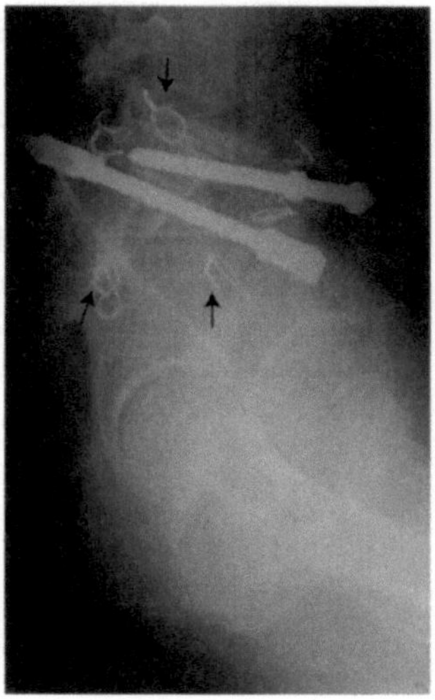

FIG. 7. Lateral view of the reconstruction (April 17, 1986)

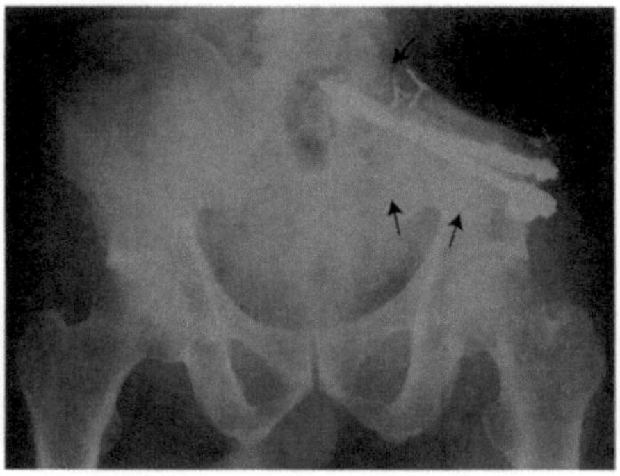

FIG. 8. AP view of the reconstructed defect in the left sacroiliac joint (March 3, 2000). The grafted segments of autogenous fibula were well homogenized and consolidated. No atrophy of the left proximal femur was noted

side on the table. The skin incision was made from the left anterior superior iliac spine, extending along the iliac crest, and curving downward at the posterior iliac spine. The resection was carried out approximately 3 cm beyond the border of the tumor, including the left sacroiliac joint. The defect in the pelvic ring was then grafted with an autogenous fibula split diagonally. The fibular grafts were placed medial-superior and lateral-inferior, and were inserted into the cancellous bone of the ilium and sacrum. A portion of the ilium was added to increase the mass of the grafted bone. The grafts were reinforced with a Harrington compression rod to generate a compressive force, and a threaded sacral bar to generate a distraction force from the lower extremity (Figs. 6 and 7).

Postoperative Course

The patient's postoperative course was uneventful, and standing and gait training were initiated 2 weeks after surgery. The patient was discharged from the hospital 2 months after surgery. A postoperative X-ray examination showed the union of the grafted bone to the ilium and sacrum.

The patient was fully ambulatory without need of any external support 6 months after surgery. He was still alive 16 years after surgery, was fully engaged in his work, and has had no sign of any recurrence of the tumor (Fig. 8).

Case 4: Recurrent Synovial Sarcoma of the Pubic Region Treated with a Wide Resection, Including the Pubic Bone and Female Genitalia in a 50-Year-Old Woman

Hideaki E. Takahashi

Summary. A recurrent synovial sarcoma occurred in the region of the labia majora, clitoris, and urethra. This tumor was treated operatively with resection of the adjacent skin, urethra, bladder, vagina, symphysis pubis, and the origins of the adductor and obturator muscles.

Key words. Synovial sarcoma, Pubis, Ileal conduit, Myocutaneous flap

Clinical History

The patient was found to have a tumor in the suprapubic region 4 years before her original admission in 1978. The tumor was diagnosed as a sarcoma, but was unclassified (Figs. 1 and 2). A wide resection of the tumor, including the skin, was performed, and the skin defect was closed with a right groin skin flap. The patient was subsequently treated with chemotherapy using adenomycin and endoxin. The final pathological diagnosis was a synovial sarcoma.

Six months before her most recent admission, the patient noticed a regrowth of the tumor. Upon admission, the local recurrence of the tumor was confirmed. The tumor was approximately 3 cm in diameter, elastic, and hard, and was deeply seated in the infrapubic region of the right labia majora, close to the clitoris and urethra. Plain radiographs revealed an osteosclerotic and partially osteolytic area in the inferior portion of the right ischium, close to the symphysis pubis (Fig. 3).

Surgical Procedure

In January 1983, the tumor was widely resected. Because of the location of the tumor, the resection included the adjacent skin, urethra, bladder, vagina, symphysis pubis, and a portion of the adductor and obturator muscles arising from the pubis (Fig. 4). With the patient in the Sims' position, an abdominal and vaginal total hysterectomy was performed, as well as a left salpingo-oophorectomy and total vaginectomy. An ileal conduit, anastomosed with the ureters bilaterally, was made, and a colostomy was performed and later closed. The defect in the peritoneum pubis was filled with free fascia lata. The defect in the abdominal wall and symphysis was closed with a vascularized free latissimus dorsi flap and a left groin flap. An additional rotation flap was

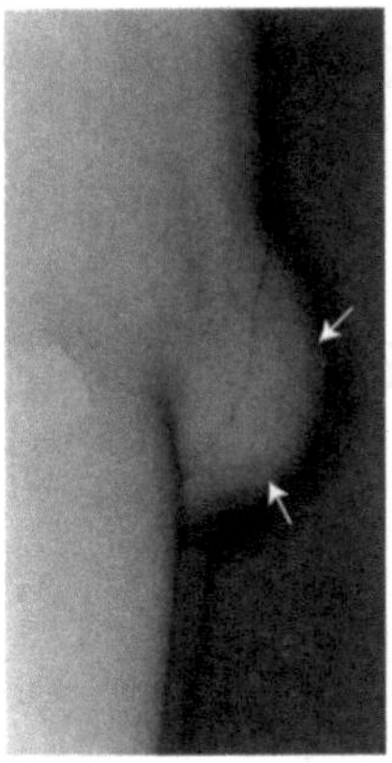

FIG. 1. Lateral view of the tumor at the time of the patient's initial surgery (August 13, 1979)

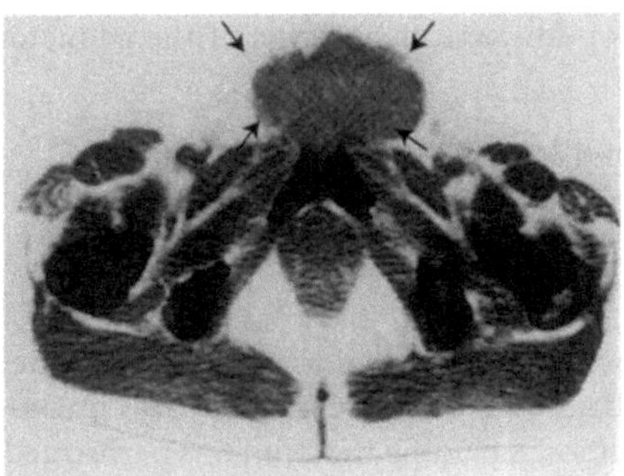

FIG. 2. Horizontal view by computed tomography showing the tumor expanding like a mushroom from the symphysis pubis (August 1979)

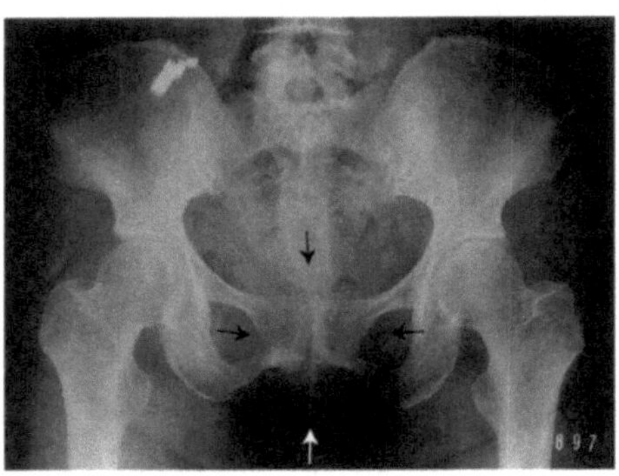

FIG. 3. Anteroposterior (AP) view of the pelvis showing the osteosclerotic lesion and partial osteolytic edge of the symphysis pubis, just beneath the recurrent tumor located at the right labia majora, close to the clitoris and urethra (October 7, 1982)

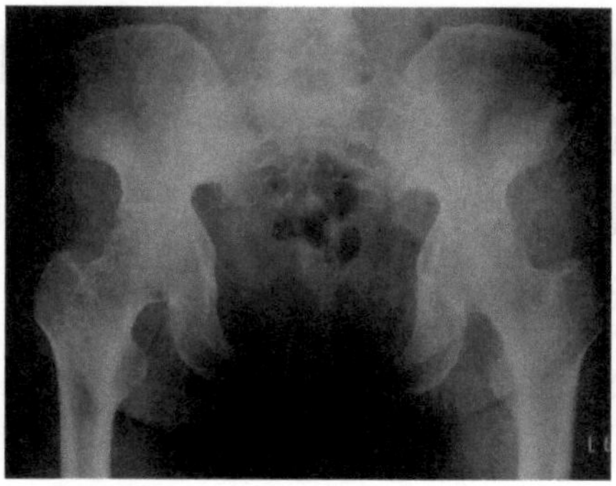

FIG. 4. AP view of the pelvis on March 16, 1995. The patient could walk without the use of any external support, although her bilateral pubic rami were defective

used to treat necrosis of the tip of the groin flap. An additional course of chemotherapy using adenomycin was administered postoperatively.

Postoperative Course

Six months after the wide resection surgery, a partial lobectomy was performed for a right pulmonary metastasis. A partial lobectomy for a left pulmonary metastasis was performed 13 months after the wide resection surgery. The patient received a course of chemotherapy with cyclophosphamide and endoxin.

The patient is still alive and generally healthy 17 years after the wide resection surgery. There has been no evidence of any local recurrence of the tumor, or further pulmonary metastasis. She is fully ambulatory and works as a housewife. The function of the ileal conduit is uneventful. The possibility of a reconstruction of the vagina was discussed after the wide resection surgery, but the patient did not want additional surgery at that time.

Discussion

A synovial sarcoma is a malignant soft tissue sarcoma that accounts for 6%–10% of all soft tissue tumors. It is the fourth most common malignant soft tissue tumor, following fibrohistiocytoma, liposarcoma, and rabdomyosarcoma. The tumor was deeply seated and located on the symphysis pubis. Because of its location and the high probability of recurrence, a wide resection of the tumor was made, including the urethra and vagina. Reconstruction using an ileal conduit was performed. After wide resection of the pubic region, the patient was found to have pulmonary metastases, which were treated with a bilateral lobectomy.

Case 5: Wide Resection of a Large Chondrosarcoma of the Ilium and Reconstruction of the Pelvic Ring in a 55-Year-Old Man

Yoshiya Inoue

Summary. To prevent postoperative wound complications after the resection of large iliac tumors, it is better to preserve the main trunk of the internal iliac artery, and to ligate each of the affected branches separately, rather than ligating all of the branches at the base.

Key words. Tumor, Pelvis, Fusion, Reconstruction, Chondrosarcoma

Clinical History

The patient presented with a 5-year history of a tumor growing in the left buttock. Plain radiography, a computed tomography scan, and magnetic resonance images indicated that a cartilaginous tumor was located outside the left iliac wing, and had wide contact with the ilium, hip joint capsule, and greater trochanter (Figs. 1–3).

Surgical Procedure

The patient was anesthetized and placed in the right lateral position. Routine scrubbing and sterile draping were performed, leaving the left lower extremity free.

Incisions were made which encircled a region of thinned skin over the tumor in the left buttock, as shown in Fig. 4. The abdominal muscles were divided at a level several centimeters medial to the tumor, along the iliac crest. The retroperitoneal space was entered, and the iliacus muscle was transected near its origin. The sartorius and rectus femoris muscles were transected at a level near their origins. The lateral femoral cutaneous nerve was also divided. At the left wall of the small pelvic cavity, the iliolumbar artery and superior gluteal artery, and their accompanying veins, were clipped and divided. The anterior aspect of the left sacroiliac joint was exposed.

With the patient in a semiprone position, the region of the greater trochanter was exposed. An osteotomy was made through the greater trochanter and into the hip joint. The gluteus maximus muscle was transected close to its femoral insertion. The hip joint was dislocated, and another osteotomy was made through the acetabulum, and extended through both anterior and posterior columns (Fig. 5). Since most of the acetabulum and femoral head could be preserved, it was decided to reconstruct the pelvic ring and fuse the hip, rather than fuse the femoral head to the sacrum. From

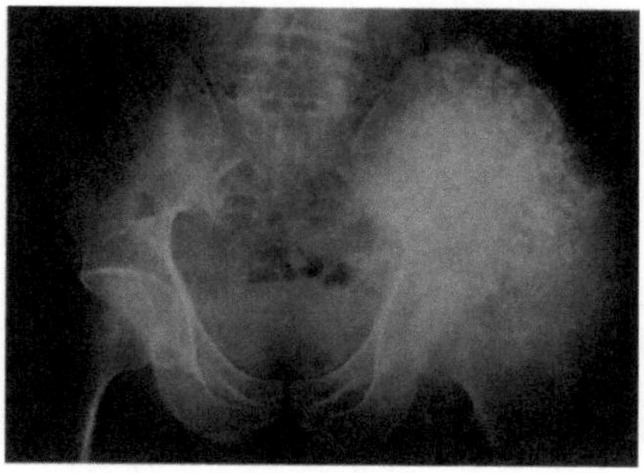

FIG. 1. Plain radiograph showing a large calcified tumor of the left ilium

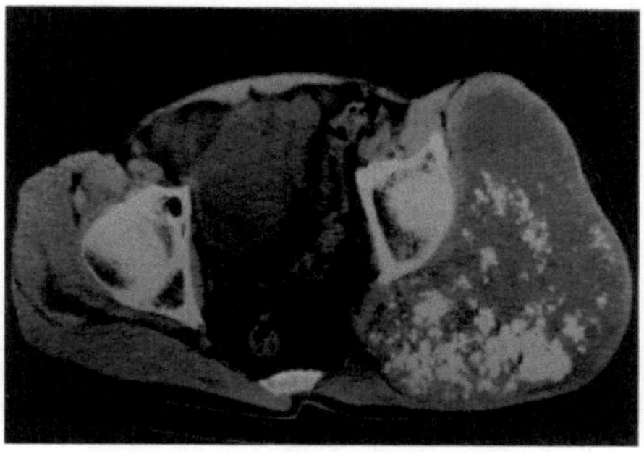

FIG. 2. Computed tomography scan showing the mineralized large tumor involving the top of the hip joint

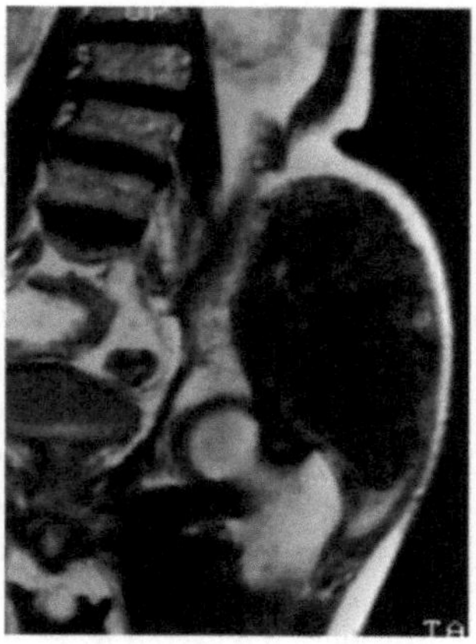

FIG. 3. Frontal magnetic resonance image showing the tumor without the involvement of the hip joint

the anterior aspect of the sacroiliac joint, a third osteotomy was made halfway through the left sacroiliac joint. From the posterior aspect of the sacroiliac joint, the gluteus maximus muscle was transected, and an osteotomy was made through the remainder of the sacroiliac joint to complete the disarticulation (Fig. 5). The caudal portion of the gluteus maximus muscle was transected. The underlying piriformis muscle was also transected, and the sacrospinous ligament was divided. The entire ilium, includ-

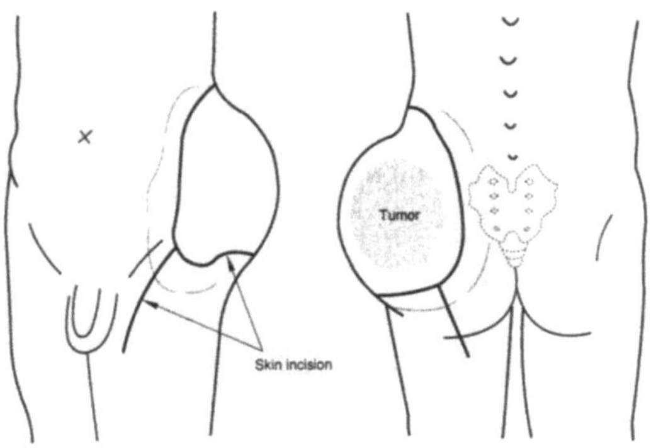

FIG. 4. Anterior and posterior skin incisions

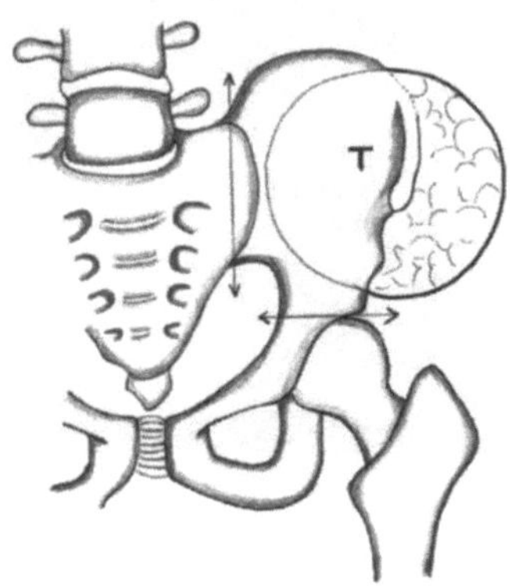

FIG. 5. The osteotomy lines, indicated by the double-headed arrows

ing the tumor, was then removed (Fig. 5). After thorough saline irrigation of the wound, the reconstructive procedures were initiated.

The articular cartilage of the remaining portion of the acetabulum was excised, and the subchondral bone was decorticated. The superiomedial portion of the articular cartilage of the femoral head, which came into contact with the remaining cartilage of the acetabulum, was removed, and the subchondral bone was decorticated. The femoral head was fixed to the acetabulum and ischium with screws in a position with 30° of flexion, 0° of abduction, and 0° of rotation (Fig. 6). The defect between the sacrum and the femoral head was bridged with two struts of nonvascularized fibula harvested from the ipsilateral leg. The distal ends of these struts were inserted into the femoral head, while the other ends were fixed to the sacrum with screws. Bone chips were harvested from the great trochanter and grafted to the fusion site (Fig. 6). The remaining muscles were reapproximated and sutured. The skin defect on the buttock was covered with a free latissimus dorsi myocutaneous flap. The flap's vascular pedicle was sutured to the inferior gluteal artery and vein.

It is important to avoid postoperative ischemic changes in the soft tissues around the pelvis. Such ischemia can easily lead to deep infection, particularly when the tumor is large. In order to prevent ischemia, it is much better to preserve the main trunk of the internal iliac artery, and to ligate each of the affected branches separately, rather than ligating all of the branches together at the base. If the gluteal flap is impor-

FIG. 6. Schematic diagram of the reconstruction

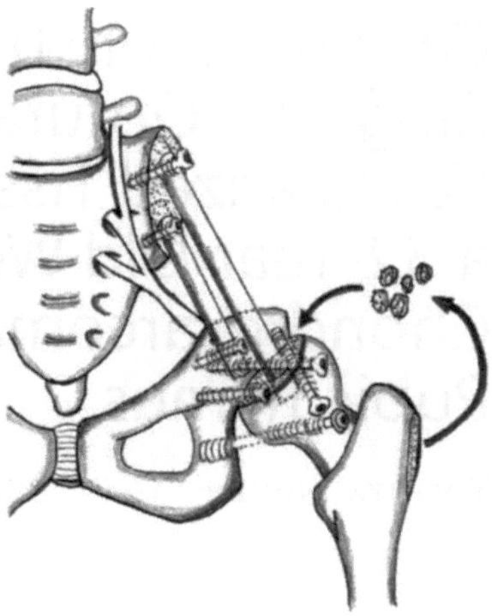

tant in any particular case, blood circulation from at least one of the superior or inferior gluteal arteries is critical.

Summary of Surgical Procedure

—Resection: subtotal wide resection of the left hemipelvis.
—Reconstruction: the left portion of the pelvic ring was reconstructed with the ipsilateral fibula, and covered with a free latissimus dorsi myocutaneous flap.
—Procedure: wide excision.
—Operative time: 13 h 20 min.
—Total blood loss: 1100 ml.
—Blood transfusion: 800 ml.

Case 6: Reconstruction of the Pelvic Ring and Obturator Nerve with Vascularized Tissue Transfers in a 32-Year-Old Woman with a Chondrosarcoma of the Inferior Pubic Ramus

Yoshiya Inoue

Summary. The obturator artery and vein should be clearly identified and ligated near their entrance and exit from the tumor. Otherwise, accidental laceration of these vessels during tumor resection may lead to a large loss of blood that could become uncontrollable.

Key words. Tumor, Pelvis, Vascularized fibula, Nerve

Clinical History

The patient presented with a 10-month history of a growing mass in the left pubic region. Plain radiographs and a computed tomography scan revealed a massive cartilaginous tumor arising from the inferior pubic ramus (Fig. 1). The tumor originated from the left inferior pubic ramus, and extended into the pubic body.

Surgical Procedure

The patient was anesthetized and placed in the prone position. The left lower limb was scrubbed and draped in the usual manner. Under the control of an Esmarch rubber bandage and an air tourniquet, a straight longitudinal skin incision was made along the fibula. The lateral sural nerve and fibula were harvested, along with their mutual feeder peroneal vessels (Fig. 2). The tourniquet was released, and the wound was closed after bleeding was controlled. An elastic bandage was applied to the wound on the lower leg.

The patient was turned and placed in the lithotomy position, and the necessary scrubbing and sterile draping were performed. The tumor mass was palpated subcutaneously and outlined on the skin with a surgical pen. The skin incision was made as shown in Fig. 3. The osteotomy lines were planned along the superior pubic ramus, through the pubic body, and just medial to the sciatic tubercle (Fig. 4). The intrapelvic space was opened by splitting the aponeurosis of the obliquus externus muscle just medial to the superficial inguinal ring. The proximal portions of the obturator artery

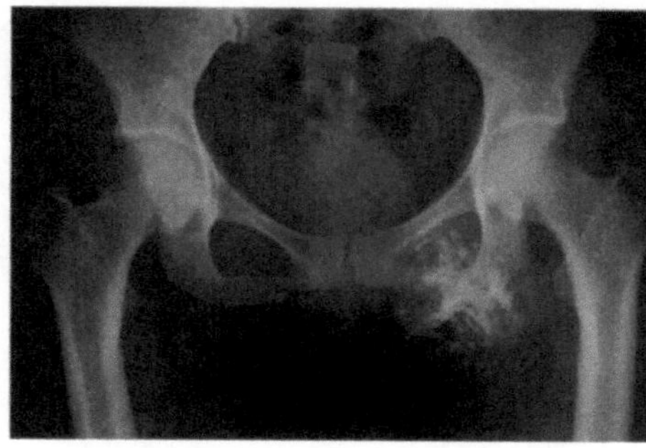

FIG. 1. Radiograph showing a cartilaginous tumor arising from the inferior pubic ramus

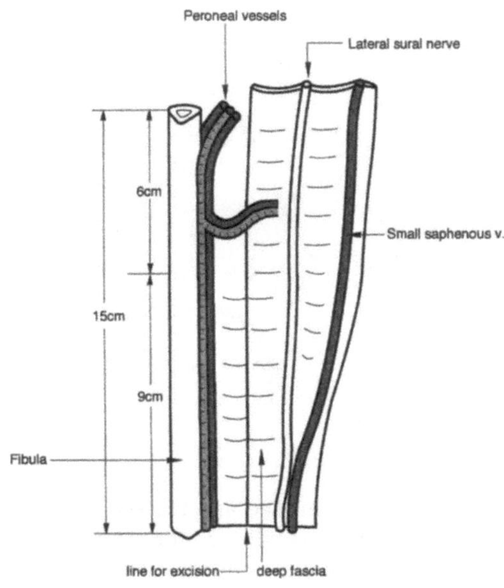

FIG. 2. Schematic diagram of the harvested vascularized fibula and the sural nerve

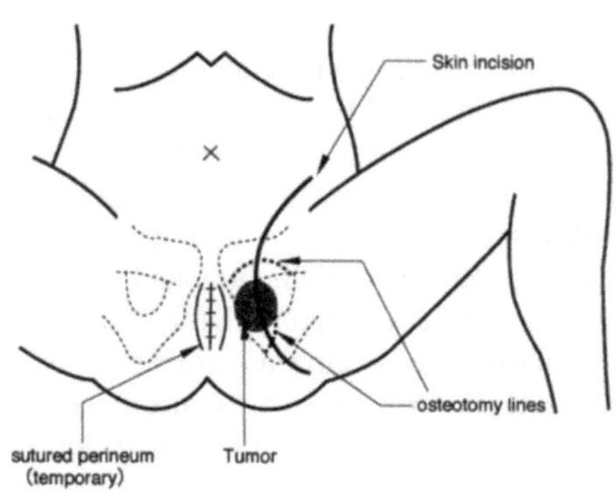

FIG. 3. Skin incision

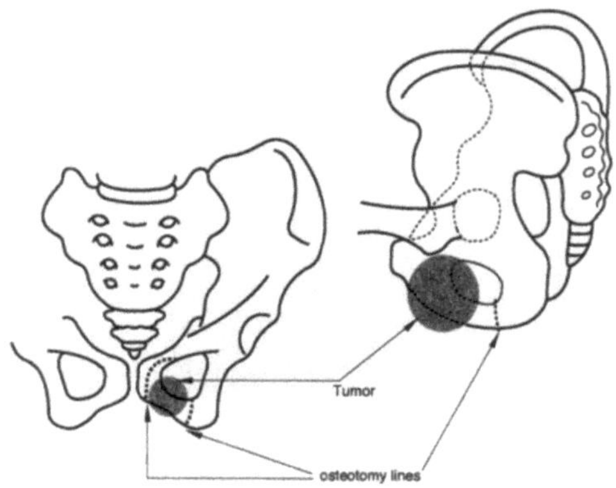

FIG. 4. Schematic diagram of the osteotomy lines

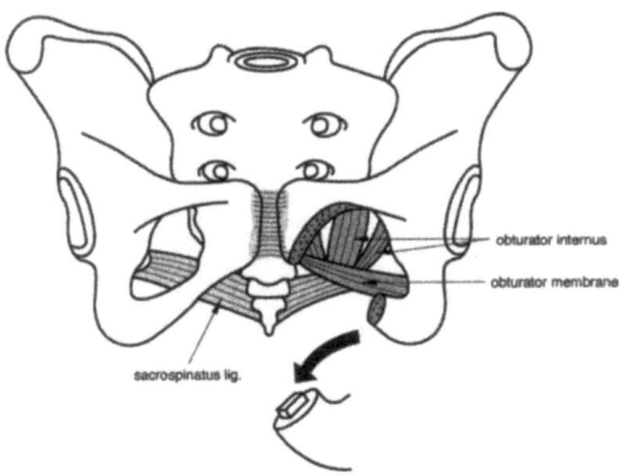

FIG. 5. Schematic diagram of the pelvis after the tumoral resection

and vein were identified and marked in the intrapelvic area with a vessel loop. The same procedure was followed for the obturator nerve. The obturator artery and vein were clipped and cut simultaneously, and the obturator nerve was cut. In the distal extrapelvic site, the anterior and posterior divisions of the obturator nerve were identified and sharply cut. The symphysis pubis was identified, and its bony surface was exposed. The corpus and superior ramus of the pubic bone were cut with a wide margin, including a portion of the muscle belly of the adductor group (Figs. 4 and 5). The vascularized fibula, which had been harvested in advance, and the stump of the residual pubic bone were trimmed to fit together, and were fixed to each other with an A–O miniscrew (Fig. 6). The peroneal artery and vein were sutured to the inferior epigastric artery and vein (Fig. 7). The lateral sural nerve had been harvested in advance, along with the attached deep fascia, which contained the small saphenous vein and a feeding artery that communicated with the peroneal artery. The harvested small saphenous vein was sutured to the concomitant vein of the obturator artery, and the lateral sural nerve was sutured to the proximal stump of the obturator nerve, and to the distal stumps of the obturator nerve's anterior and posterior divisions. The remaining reflected muscles were advanced and reattached to the pubic bone using a drilled hole with a frog position (Fig. 7). The wound was closed after irrigation. A

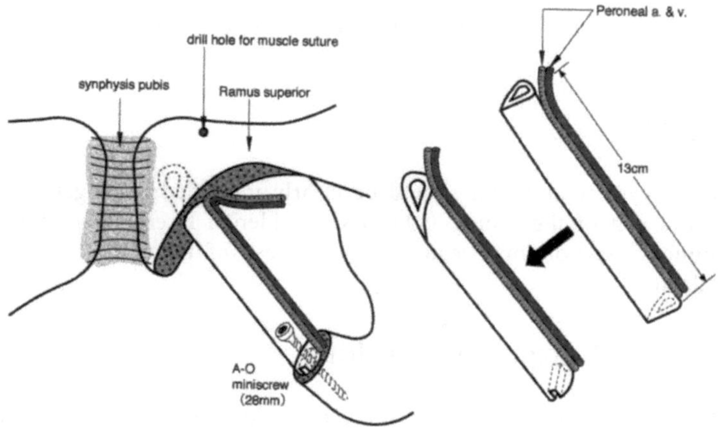

FIG. 6. Schematic diagram of the fibula graft

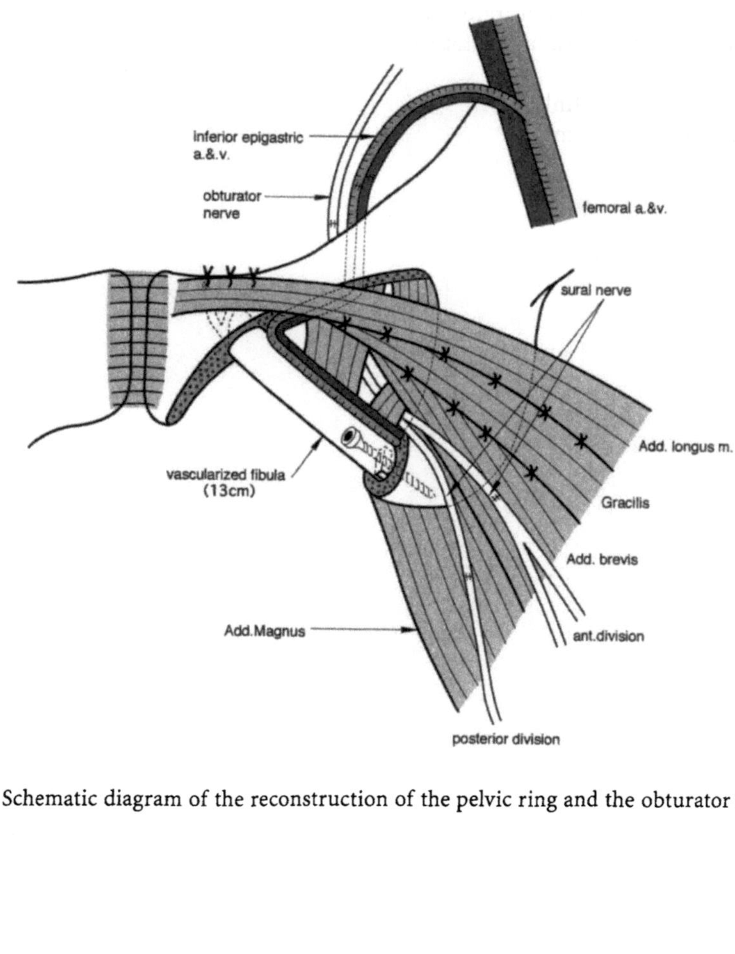

FIG. 7. Schematic diagram of the reconstruction of the pelvic ring and the obturator nerve

suction drain was placed in the wound, and a Penrose drain was placed in the retroperitoneal space.

Discussion

The obturator artery and vein should be clearly identified and ligated near their entrance and exit of the tumor. Otherwise, accidental laceration of these vessels during tumor resection may lead to a large loss of blood that could become uncontrollable.

Summary of Surgical Procedure

—Resection: wide resection of the tumor, along with the left obturator artery, vein, and nerve.
—Reconstruction: the left inferior pubic ramus was reconstructed with an ipsilateral vascularized fibular graft. A vascularized sural nerve graft was used to compensate for the removal of the obturator nerve.
—Procedure: wide excision. Operative time:
—10 h 31 min.
—Total blood loss: 530 ml.
—Blood transfusion: 0 ml.

Case 7: Partial Resection of the Sacrum and Reconstruction of the Pelvic Ring in a 41-Year-Old Man with a Giant Cell Tumor of the Sacrum

Yoshiya Inoue

Summary. Intermittent clamping of the abdominal aorta may be effective for the control of massive intraoperative bleeding in pelvic surgery.

Key words. Tumor, Pelvis, Aorta, Clamp, Declamp

Clinical History

The patient presented with a 3-month history of pain in the left buttock. Plain radiography, a computed tomography scan, and magnetic resonance imaging showed that an osteolytic lesion occupied almost the entire sacrum (Figs. 1–3). The anterior cortex of the lower sacrum was completely destroyed, and the tumor was covered by the periosteum and fascia of the anterior sacrococcygeal muscle. An open biopsy revealed a giant cell tumor of the bone.

Surgical Procedure

After induction by general anesthesia, the patient was placed in the right lateral position, and was prepared for surgery by scrubbing and draping in the usual manner.

A J-shaped incision was made for a pararectal approach. The left inferior epigastric artery was ligated and cut. The left rectus abdominis muscle was detached from its pubic insertion, and the retroperitoneal space was entered. A retractor was used to expose the tumor. The tumor was slightly shifted to the left, and protruded anteriorly. The abdominal aorta, proximal to the fourth lumbar arteries, was temporarily clamped using a Fogarty clamp (Fig. 4). The median sacral artery, left lateral sacral artery, and superior gluteal artery were ligated and cut. The right iliolumbar artery and lateral sacral artery, together with their concomitant veins, were also ligated and cut (Fig. 5). The left internal iliac vein was doubly ligated and cut, and the osteotomy surface of the sacrum was exposed (Fig. 4). The intact area of the anterior sacral cortex was osteotomized as shown in Figs. 6 and 7. The aorta was then declamped after packing sufficient gauze into the cavity.

A second longitudinal skin incision was made for a posterior approach, and included the biopsy scar with a wide margin. The posterior surface of the sacrum was

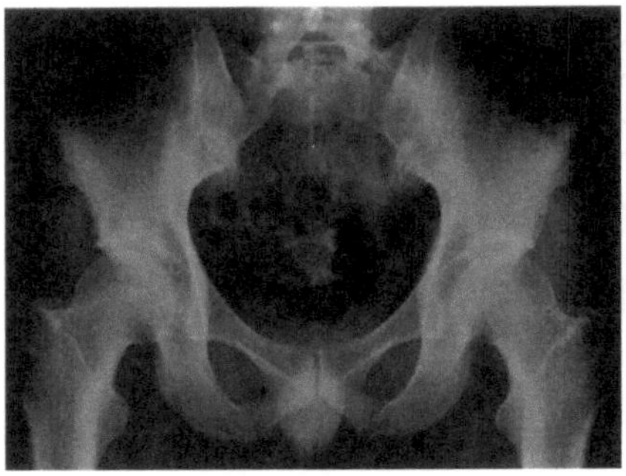

FIG. 1. Radiograph showing osteolytic changes in the sacrum

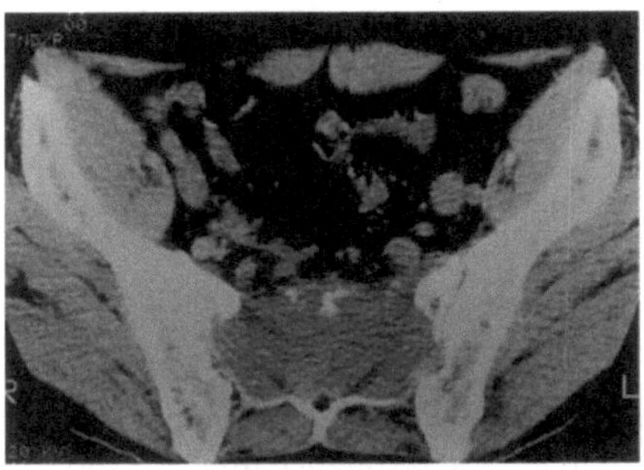

FIG. 2. Computed tomography scan showing the osteolytic lesion of the sacrum

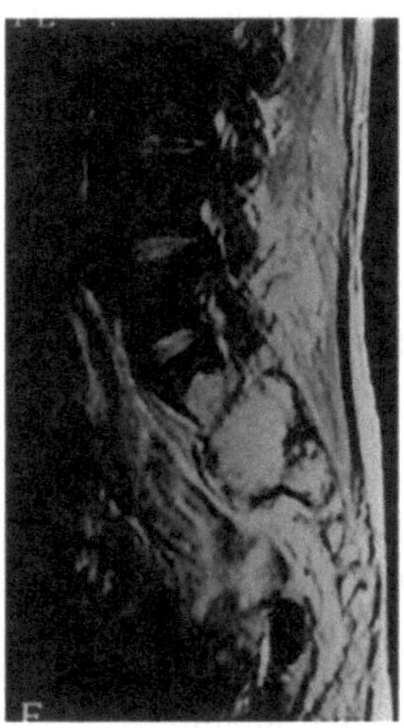

FIG. 3. Sagittal magnetic resonance image showing that the sacral tumor occupied almost the entire sacrum

exposed by reflecting the gluteus maximus and sacrococcygeal muscles (Fig. 7). The distal osteotomy line passed through S4/S5, and the proximal osteotomy line passed through S1/S2. Further curettage was required in the proximal cavity. The aorta was again clamped. The S1 cavity was thoroughly curetted using an air drill and bone curettes. The tumor mass, attached around the sacral nerve roots, was aspirated by CUSA, and the right S4 and S5 roots, and the left S3, S4, and S5 roots were all

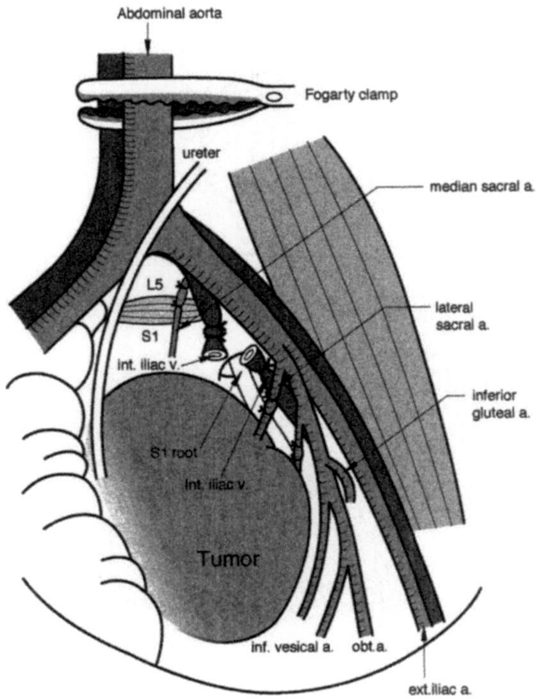

FIG. 4. Schematic diagram of the temporary clamping of the aorta

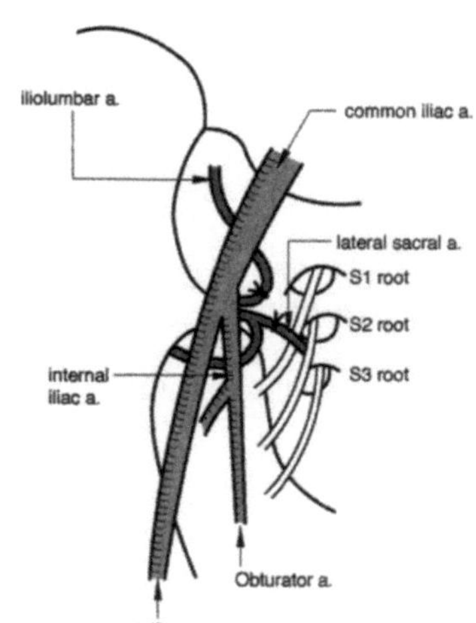

FIG. 5. Schematic diagram of the ligations of the iliolumbar arteries

sacrificed. The right S1, S2, and S3 nerve roots, and the left S1 and S2 roots were all preserved.

After declamping the aorta, an appropriate 22-cm length of fibula was harvested subperiosteally from the left leg. The fibula was divided into 9-cm and 13-cm struts for bone grafting. The smaller fibular bone graft was placed transversely, interdigitating into both sides of the ilium marrow cavity (Fig. 8). The larger bone graft was

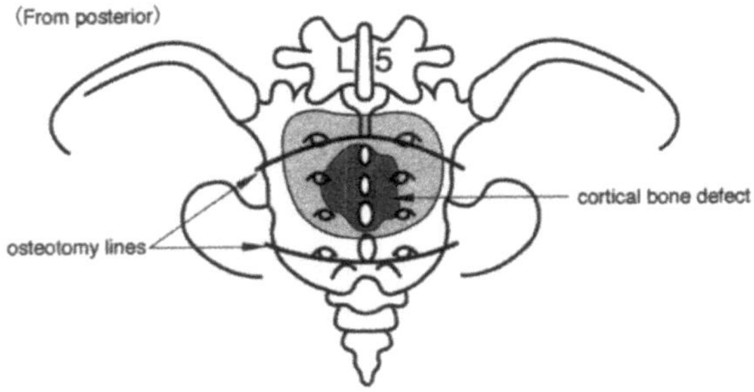

FIG. 6. Schematic diagram of the osteotomy lines

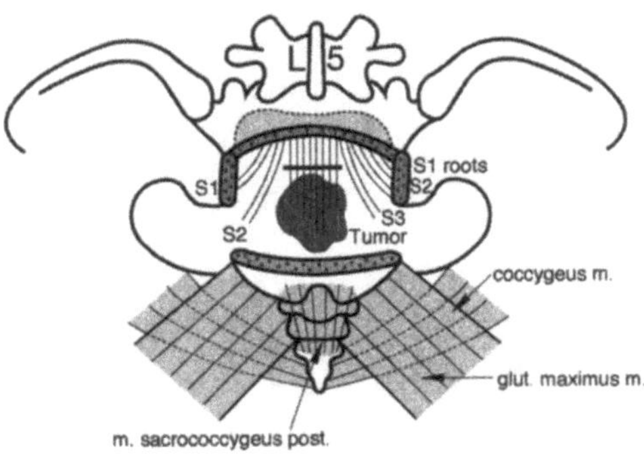

FIG. 7. Schematic diagram of the osteotomy lines

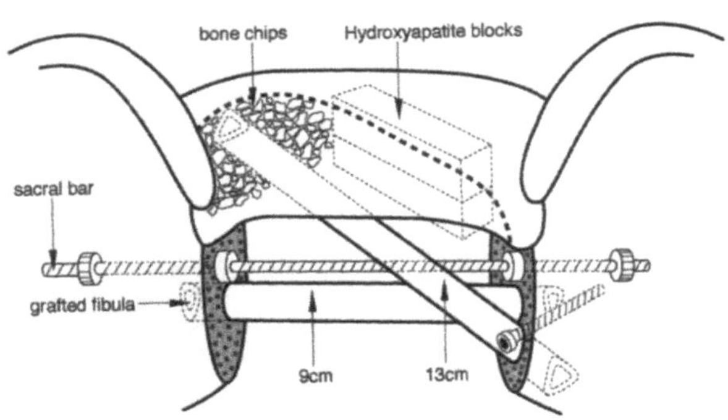

FIG. 8. Schematic diagram of the reconstruction of the pelvic ring and the bone graft

placed in an oblique orientation, and was fixed to the ilium with an A–O cortical screw. The left side of the sacral cavity was partially filled with bone chips harvested from the stumps of the ilium. Two blocks of hydroxyapatite were packed into the right side of the sacral cavity. Finally, both sides of the ilium were connected by a sacral bar with a compression force. The pelvic ring was then assessed and found to have good stability. After placing a drainage tube, the wounds were closed in layers. The post-operative anterior–posterior radiograph is shown in Fig. 9.

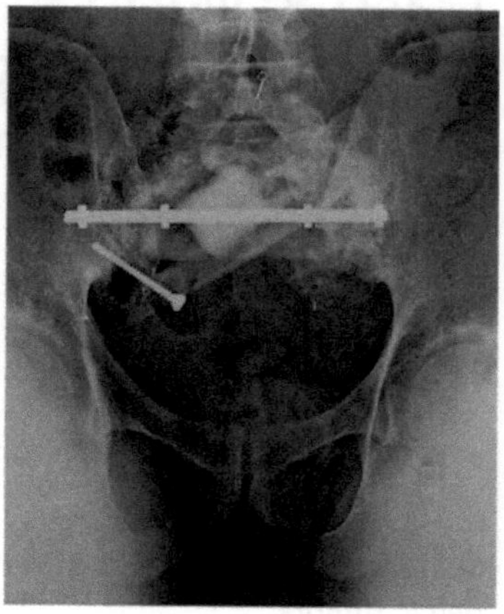

FIG. 9. Postoperative radiograph

Discussion

If the sacrum was amputated at the S1/S2 level, the bilateral S2, S3, and S4 nerve roots would all need to be sacrificed, and yet the surgical margin would be intralesional. In such cases, vesicourinary disturbance would be unavoidable. A giant cell tumor has a locally aggressive nature, but is not malignant. In the present case, we attempted to preserve as many sacral nerve roots as possible, even though the proximal surgical margin was intralesional. Postoperative radiation was required. When the surgical procedure is intralesional, blood loss is much greater than with a wide excision. Because of this, the intermittent clamping of the abdominal aorta, at a level proximal to the iliolumbar arteries, is very effective in controlling blood loss. In such a situation, the operator must take care not to mistake the bifurcation of the external and internal iliac arteries for the bifurcation of the abdominal aorta.

Summary of Surgical Procedure

—Resection: sacrum.
—Reconstruction: pelvic ring.
—Procedure: intralesional excision, and reconstruction of the pelvic ring with fibular strut grafts and a sacral bar.
—Operative time: 13 h 59 min.
—Total blood loss: 6670 ml.
—Blood transfusion: 6350 ml.
—Point of interest: intermittent clamping of the abdominal aorta (repeated every 2 h).

Case 8: Wide Excision of a Metastatic Renal Cell Carcinoma of the Ilium in a 54-Year-Old Woman

Yoshiya Inoue

Summary. Preoperative transarterial embolization is effective for hypervascular pelvic tumors.

Key words. Embolization, Cancer, Metastasis, Tumor, Pelvis

Clinical History

A patient with a history of renal cell cancer presented with left buttock pain. A computed tomography scan revealed a large osteolytic tumor of the left ilium (Fig. 1). Preoperative transarterial embolization was performed. In this particular case, preoperative transarterial embolization should be helpful in reducing intraoperative blood loss.

Surgical Procedure

After induction by general anesthesia, the patient was placed in the right lateral position. The operative fields for the pelvis and lower limb (to harvest a fibular graft, if necessary) were scrubbed and draped in the usual fashion.

A skin incision was made along the left inguinal band anteriorly, and along the iliac crest toward the posterior superior iliac spine. The internal and external obliquus abdominis muscles and transverse abdominal muscle were cut with an electrocoagulator near their myotendinous junctions just inside the left iliac wing. The retroperitoneal space was then entered. The psoas muscle was retracted laterally to expose the segmental arteries of L4 and L5. The segmental artery of L4 was larger in diameter, and was ligated and cut. The segmental artery of L5 was coagulated because it was smaller. The iliaca interna artery was then doubly ligated. The tumor was palpated over the iliacus muscle, and was found to have a clear margin (Fig. 2). The inner surface of the left iliac wing was exposed with a 1.5-cm margin from the edge of the tumor.

A posterior skin incision was then made. The gluteus maximus muscle was detached from the left iliac crest after it was found that there were no adhesions between it and the gluteus medius muscle, which in turn covered the tumor. The tumor did not extend to the gluteus minimus muscle. The gluteus medius muscle was

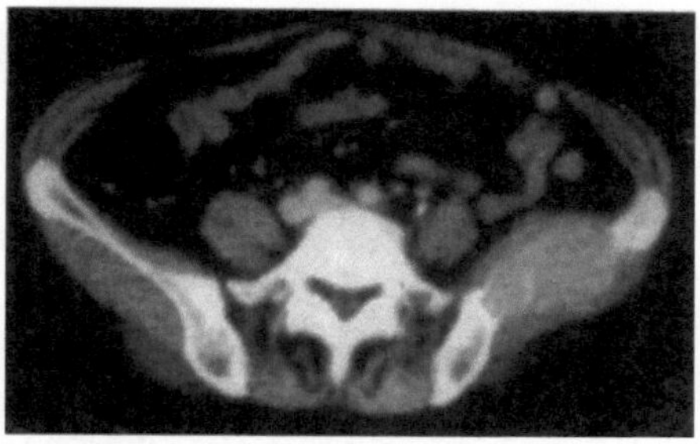

FIG. 1. Computed tomography scan showing metastatic renal cell cancer of the ilium

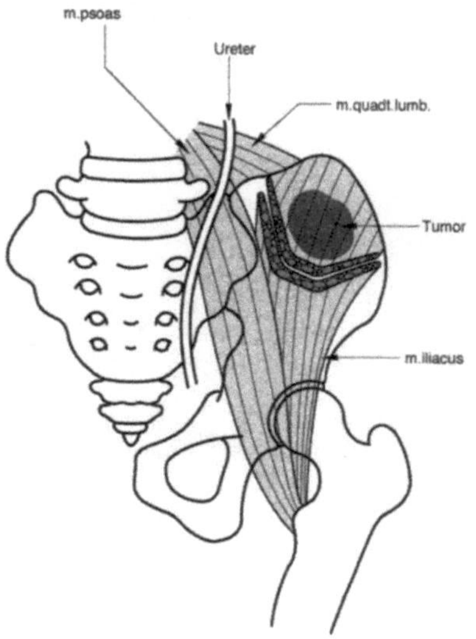

FIG. 2. Schematic diagram of the excised area

divided with the electrocoagulator to expose the outer surface of the left iliac wing with a 1.5-cm margin (Fig. 3). An osteotomy of the ilium was initiated with an osteotome from its inner surface to its outer surface. The tumor was resected with the iliacus and gluteus medius muscles (Figs. 2 and 3). Each stump of the abdominal muscles and the gluteus maximus muscle were sutured together after the fixation of an intact part of the resected ilium to the ilium corner with two K-wires (Fig. 4).

Discussion

When a tumor markedly protrudes into the pelvic cavity, the bifurcation of the external and internal iliac arteries is similar to the bifurcation of the abdominal aorta. Moreover, it is sometimes difficult to identify the ureter on the affected side. The surgeon should have a clear understanding of the abnormal anatomy from multiple preoperative images. Even though the ligation of the internal iliac artery is unavoidable, it is preferable to preserve the internal iliac vein in order to minimize blood loss (Figs. 3 and 4).

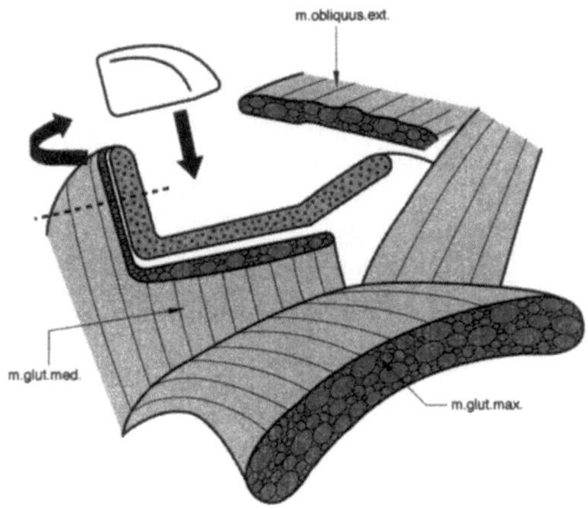

FIG. 3. Schematic diagram of the resection of the ilium

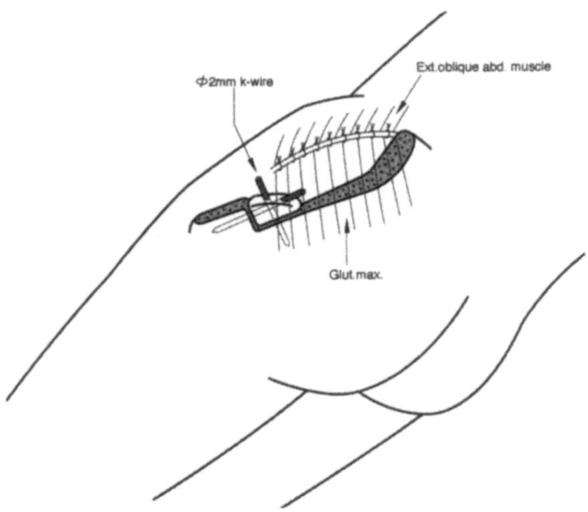

FIG. 4. Schematic diagram of the wound closure and iliac bone graft

Summary of Surgical Procedure

—Resection: left iliac wing with surrounding musculature.
—Reconstruction: partial left iliac wing using a portion of the resected ilium.
—Procedure: wide excision.
—Operative time: 3h.
—Total blood loss: 831ml.
—Blood transfusion: 800ml.

Case 9: Resection of a Chordoma of the Sacrum in a 40-Year-Old Man

Tetsuo Hotta

Summary. A 40-year-old man with a stage II-B chordoma of the sacrum received an en-bloc resection of the tumor with a posterior approach.

Key words. Chordoma, Sacral amputation, Posterior approach, Wide excision, Vesicorectal disfunction

Clinical History

In 1993, the patient experienced pain in the sacral region. In August 1996, he was admitted to a city hospital for an evaluation of a suspected IgA nephropathy. An unexpected sacral tumor was found by the computed tomography scan (Fig. 1). The patient was referred to Niigata University Hospital in September 1996. Fine-needle aspiration cytology from the mass in the paravertebral muscle suggested a chordoma. Magnetic resonance imaging findings were compatible with the diagnosis of a chordoma (Fig. 2). It was decided to perform an en bloc resection with a posterior approach without an open biopsy.

Surgical Procedure

Routine preoperative preparations for a sacrectomy were performed (see Chap. 4). The surgical procedure is described in detail in Chap. 5. by T. Hotta, this volume. A reverse Y-shaped skin incision was made to obtain a wide exposure of both sides of the sacrum and sciatic notch. The tumor extended posteriorly on the lamina, and was covered by the gluteus maximus muscle. The muscle was transected with a 1-cm margin using a bipolar electrocoagulator. A laminectomy of S2 was performed, and the roots below S3 were sharply severed. The sacrotuberous and sacrospinous ligaments were carefully cut. The piriformis muscle was also transected. The sciatic nerve and gluteal vessels were identified and protected. The anterior surface of the sacrum was bluntly dissected at the level of the osteotomy, between S2 and S3. A sponge was introduced into the sciatic notch and passed through to the opposite notch. An osteotomy was performed with an osteotome. The stump was reflected distally, and the rectum was easily freed from the tumor beyond the loose areolar tissue. Wide excision was completely satisfactory (Fig. 3). The defect was covered with marlex mesh.

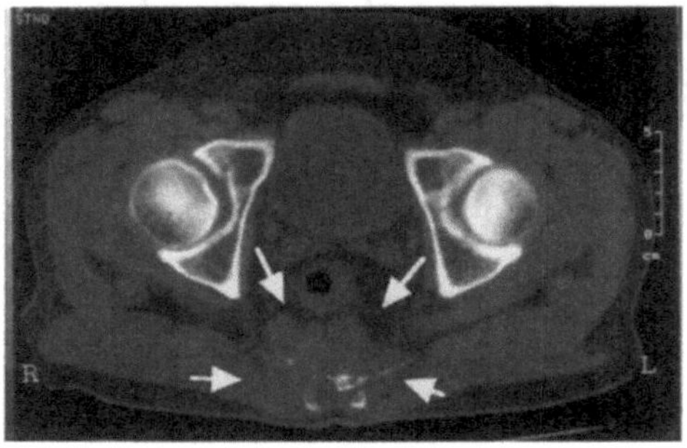

Fig. 1. A computerized axial tomography scan revealed an unexpected sacral tumor (*arrows*)

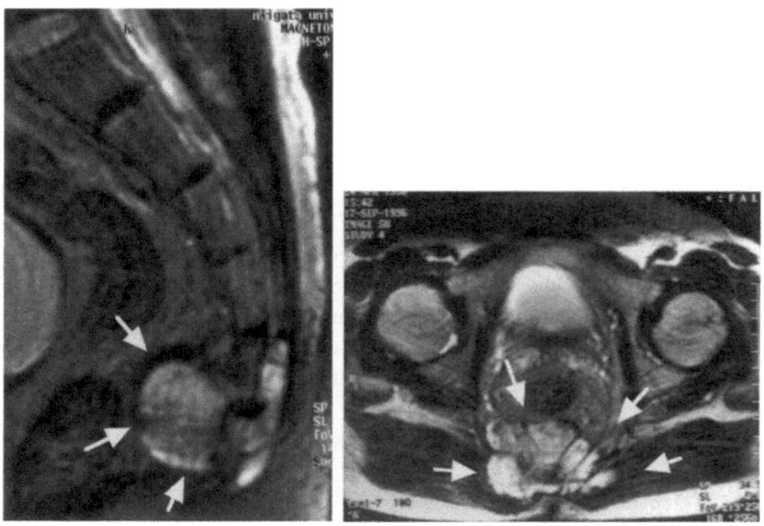

a b

Fig. 2. T2-weighted magnetic resonance image. **a** The sagittal view shows a presacral high-intensity tumor (*arrows*). **b** Tumor invasion into the gluteus maximus muscle (*arrows*) is evident in the axial view

The wound was primarily closed without packing the dead space. There were no complications. Blood loss was 800 ml, and 800 ml of autogenous blood was transfused into the patient. The total operative time was 4 h. Postoperative X-ray film shows the level of amputation, S2/3 (Fig. 4).

It is important to make the proximal osteotomy first, and then the dissection between the rectum and the sacrum can be accomplished by reflecting the tumor-bearing sacrum. The dissection should be done from the proximal to the distal side.

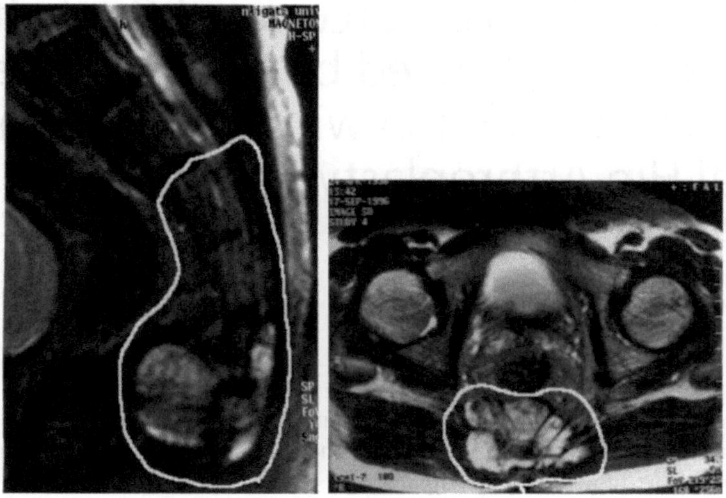

a b

FIG. 3. Surgical margin. **a** The sagittal margin was between S2 and S3. **b** The axial margin was 1 cm from the tumor

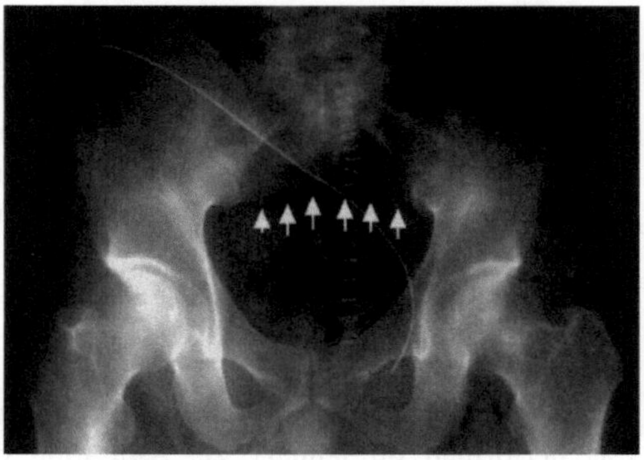

FIG. 4. Postoperative X-ray film. The sacrum below S2 was resected (*arrows*)

The S3 and lower nerve roots were sacrificed bilaterally. No additional motor weakness was observed. A slight vesicorectal disturbance appeared. Erectile deficiency and minor urinary incontinence were observed 5 years after surgery. The patient is alive and healthy 5 years after surgery, and there has been no local recurrence of the tumor or distant metastasis.

Case 10: Chondrosarcoma of the Left Acetabulum Treated by Osteotomy and Hip Reconstruction with Conventional Total Hip Arthroplasty in a 62-Year-Old Woman

Tetsuo Hotta

Summary. A female patient with a cystic lesion in her left acetabulum was diagnosed as having a chondrosarcoma. A three-dimensional osteotomy was performed for resection of the tumor. This was followed by a conventional total hip arthroplasty (THA) with bone grafting.

Key words. Chondrosarcoma, Three-dimensional osteotomy, Type II, Conventional THA, Bone graft

Clinical History

The patient experienced a dull pain in her left hip joint 2 years before admission. The pain gradually worsened, and she visited a nearby orthopedic clinic. X-ray examination showed a cystic lesion in her left acetabulum (Fig. 1). Calcification was not detected. Magnetic resonance imaging revealed extremely high intensity T2-weighted images (Fig. 2), and slightly high intensity T1-weighted images. Moderate contrast enhancement was observed. A computerized axial tomography scan showed the destruction of the anterior half of the acetabulum (Fig. 3). The patient was referred to Niigata University Hospital, and was admitted on January 14, 1998. The surgery was performed on January 26. Aspiration cytology revealed the features of a chondrosarcoma.

Preoperative planning for a three-dimensional pelvic osteotomy was performed using a paper template model of the pelvis. The aim of surgery in this particular case was to preserve the posterior column of the acetabulum. An attempt was made to avoid reconstructing the pelvic ring if at all possible. Routine preoperative preparations for a sacrectomy were made, including the cleansing of the bowel. This procedure is described in detail in Chap. 5 by T. Morita, this volume.

Surgical Procedure

The patient was placed in the right lateral position after successful induction of general anesthesia. The left pelvic girdle and lower limb were scrubbed and draped in the same manner as for a hemipelvectomy. The skin incision is shown in Fig. 4. Skin necrosis did not occur in this case. An ilioinguinal approach was made first, and

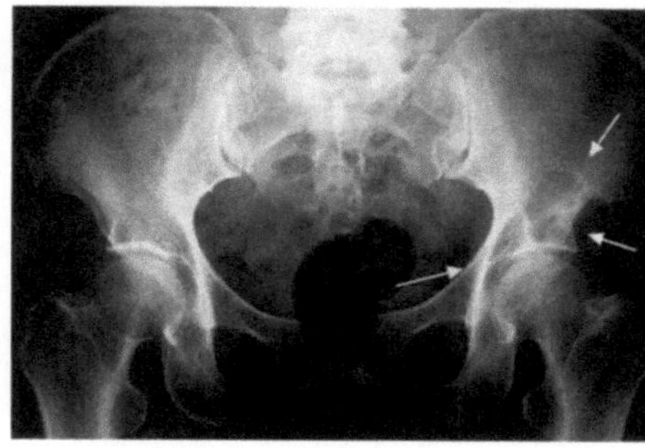

FIG. 1. Preoperative X-ray film showing a cystic lesion in the roof of the acetabulum (*arrows*)

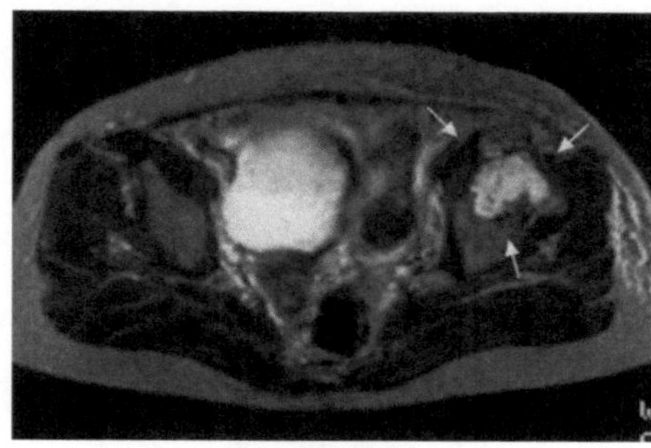

FIG. 2. T2-weighted MR image showing the high-intensity lesion (*arrows*)

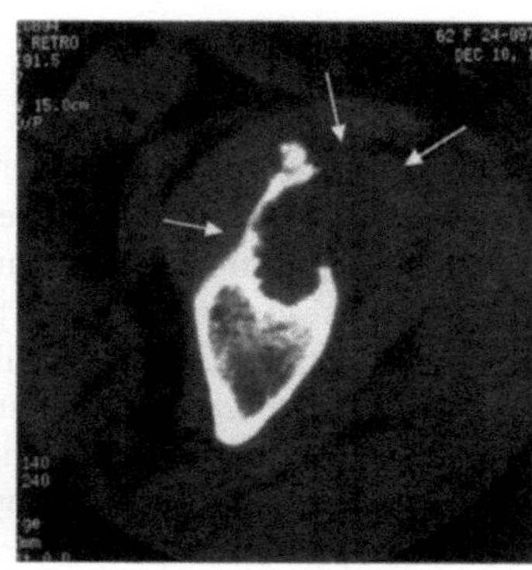

FIG. 3. Computed axial tomography scan showing the destruction of the anterior half of the acetabulum (*arrows*)

the pelvic cavity was widely exposed. It was found that the iliacus would have to be resected with the tumor, since the tumor extended out from the inner cortex of the pelvis. Because of this, identification of the external iliac artery and vein, and the internal iliac artery and vein, was carried out at this time.

A lateral approach was then made. The tumor extended mainly anteriorly, and was covered by the tensor fascia lata and gluteus minimus. The gluteus maximus was severed at its insertion, and the gluteus medius was also temporarily transected. The short rotators were severed at their femoral insertions. The posterior wall of the

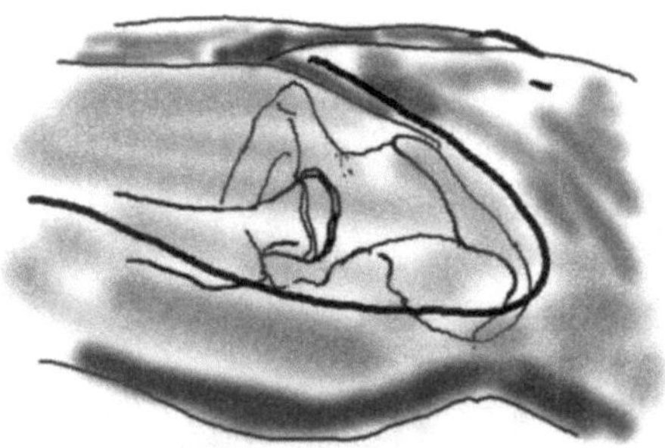

FIG. 4. Skin incision. A combined ilioinguinal and lateral femoral approach was made

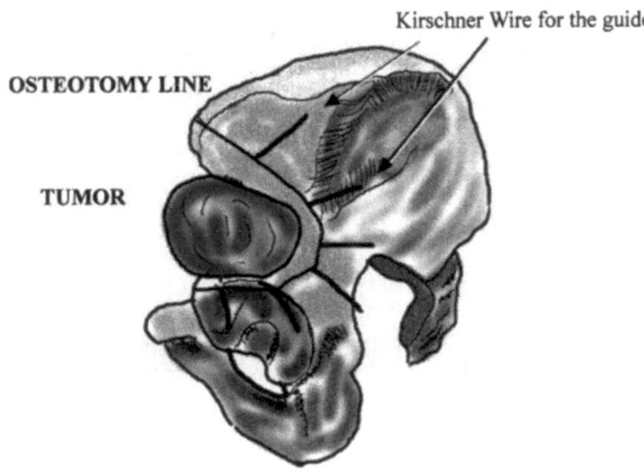

FIG. 5. A three-dimensional osteotomy line was designed, and several Kirschner wires were introduced using the line as a guide

acetabulum was exposed subperiosteally. The iliopsoas and rectus femoris were transected at the level of the lesser trochanter.

The capsule of hip joint was cut circumferentially near its femoral attachment, and the femoral head was dislocated posteriorly. There was no evidence of tumor tissue in the hip joint, and the joint cartilage of the acetabulum was intact. The femoral neck was osteotomized to accommodate a prosthesis.

Several Kirschner wires were introduced along the three-dimensional osteotomy line on the ilium, as determined by preoperative planning (Fig. 5). The osteotomy was then made with an osteotome along the path of the Kirschner wires. Unfortunately, the margin at the posterior column was not adequate. Therefore, additional resection of the stump was carried out (Fig. 6), and Pasteurization was performed with hot saline (70°C) for 20 min.

The resected femoral head was trimmed and grafted into the defect in the acetabular roof, and was fixed with two cortical screws. The acetabulum was then reamed in the usual manner. An OMNIFIT PSL (Peripheral Self-Locking) cup (Nippon Stryker, Tokyo, Japan) was implanted and fixed with screws. An OMNIFLEX femoral component (Nippon Stryker) was then implanted in the usual manner (Fig. 7). The gluteus medius and gluteus maximus muscles were repaired. The stability of the joint was insufficient, and the hip was easily dislocated. However, the hip could not be sig-

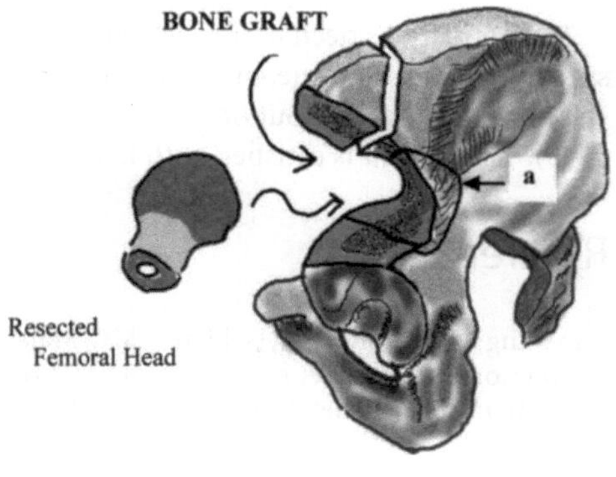

FIG. 6. Inadequate margin in the posterior column (*a*), and additional resection

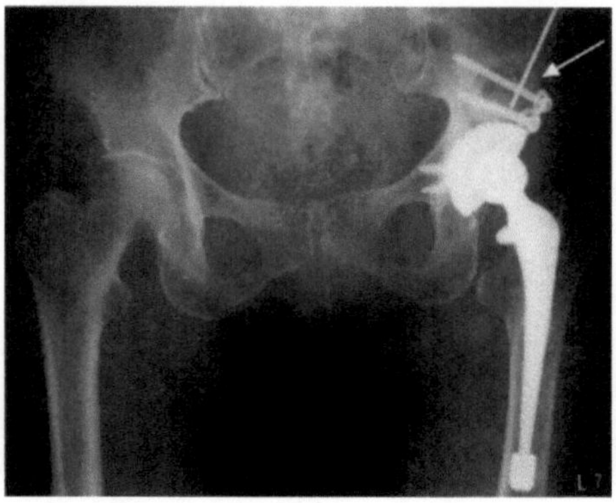

FIG. 7. Hip joint reconstruction with total hip arthroplasty. The resected femoral head was grafted into the defect in the acetabular roof, and fixed with screws (*arrow*)

nificantly reinforced in any way. The defect in the groin fascia was reconstructed with Marlex mesh, and the wound was closed.

The surgical stage in this case was I B. The surgical margin was estimated to be marginal.

Postoperative Course

The patient was given bed rest for 2 weeks. A hip spica cast was then applied for 4 weeks. Standing exercises were begun on a tilt table immediately after the cast was applied. After 2 weeks, the cast was shortened to allow free motion of the knee joint. Range-of-motion exercises of the knee joint were initiated with the patient in bed. Gait exercises were begun 7 weeks after surgery. Three months after surgery, the patient could ambulate while bearing her full weight.

Eight months after surgery, the patient complained of instability of the affected hip joint during motion in bed. Subluxation was confirmed by an image intensifier. Special rubberized short pants were designed and fabricated to stabilize the hip. The patient wore these pants all day for 6 months. She was finally able to perform the activities of daily living without the pants. Subluxation of the hip did not occur at this time.

The patient has been doing well, and has been disease-free for 37 months since the surgery. She uses a cane, but can walk short distances without it. Her limb function was rated at 24 points out of 30 points by Enneking's function score (Enneking et al. 1993). The patient is satisfied with her result. No complications occurred in this case.

Reference

Enneking WF, Dunham W, Gebhardt MC, Malawar M, Pritchard DJ (1993) A system for the functional evaluation of reconstructive procedures after surgical treatment of tumors of the musculoskeletal system. Clin Orthop 286:241–246

Case 11: Internal Hemipelvectomy and Constrained Total Hip Arthroplasty for the Treatment of Chondrosarcoma of the Acetabulum in a 52-Year-Old Woman

Tetsuo Hotta

Summary. A triple osteotomy was performed for the resection of a grade I chondrosarcoma of the left acetabulum. The hip was reconstructed by performing a constrained total hip arthroplasty using the reconstruction cup and physio-hip system (Kyocera, Kyoto, Japan).

Key words. Type II, Chondrosarcoma, Internal hemipelvectomy, Aspiration cytology, Constrained total hip arthroplasty

Clinical History

The patient had experienced pain in her left buttock for 3 years. She visited a general hospital in June 2000, and an X-ray examination revealed an osteolytic bone lesion in her left acetabulum. A metastatic bone tumor was first suspected. However, no primary cancer was detected by general and gynecological examinations. She was referred to Niigata University Hospital, and was admitted on August 11. An X-ray examination showed an irregular osteolytic lesion in the acetabulum (Fig. 1). A magnetic resonance imaging assessment showed extremely high intensity T2-weighted images (Fig. 2). An extraosseous extension of the tumor into the pelvic cavity was also evident. Laboratory data showed no abnormal findings. Fine-needle aspiration biopsy cytology was performed on August 18. The biopsy showed the features of a low-grade chondrosarcoma. Open biopsy was not performed. Surgery was performed on September 4. The patient left the hospital on October 16, but was readmitted for treatment of a seroma of her wound. She suffered from a high fever for a week, but all bacterial cultures were negative. She left the hospital again on January 31, 2001, and is currently doing very well.

Surgical Procedure

After the successful induction of general anesthesia, the patient was placed in the right lateral position on the operating table. Scrubbing and draping for a hemipelvectomy were performed in the usual manner.

A combination of ilioinguinal and modified posterior ischial approaches were made (Fig. 3). The posterior approach was carried out first, and the fasciocutaneous flap

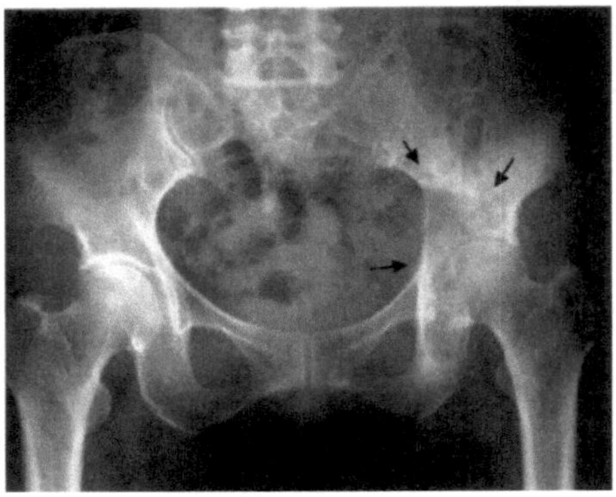

Fig. 1. Preoperative X-ray film showing an irregular osteolytic lesion in the roof of the left acetabulum (*arrows*)

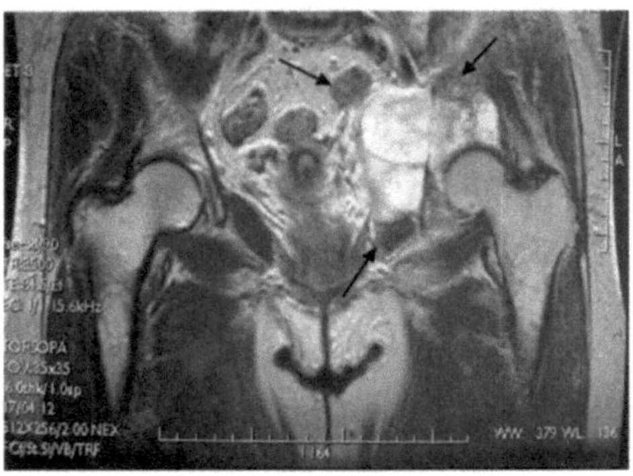

Fig. 2. T2-weighted MR image showing a high-intensity lesion (*arrows*) which extended into the pelvic cavity

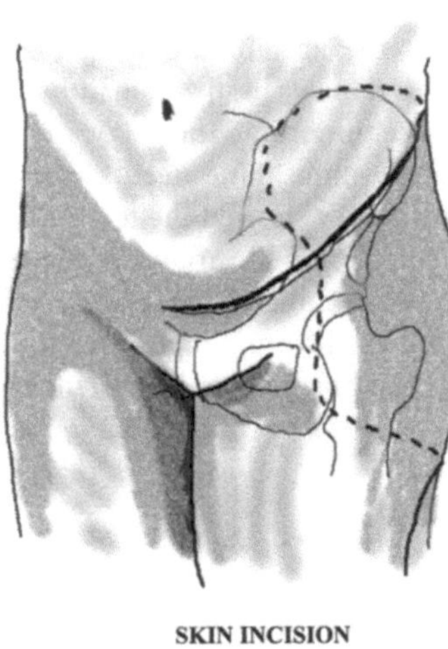

Fig. 3. Skin incision. A combination of ilioinguinal, posterior iliac, and posterior ischial approaches were used. The incision was elongated distally to expose the proximal femur

was raised. The flap was reflected anteriorly and distally to the insertion of the gluteus maximus. The insertion of the gluteus maximus was severed, and the muscle was reflected posteriorly. The sciatic nerve was easily exposed and isolated with vessel tape. The contour of the ischium was confirmed. The anterior half of the flap, together with the gluteus medius and fascia lata, was raised as a musculocutaneous flap in order to preserve the circulation of the entire flap. The flap was reflected distally to the greater trochanter. The short rotators were cut at the insertions. The medial circumflexus femoral artery was identified and severed after ligation. The origin of the rectus femoris was cut. The hip joint capsule was fully exposed.

The ilioinguinal approach was then made. The abdominal muscles were carefully severed in line. The deep circumflexus iliac artery was ligated and severed. The femoral nerve was identified at the iliac fossa, and was dissected distally. There was severe adhesion of the nerve in the inguinal region. The femoral vessels were also difficult to dissect. The lateral circumflexus femoral artery, which was thought to be the main blood supply of the posterior flap, was successfully preserved. However, the femoral vein was injured during dissection. It was sutured and repaired. Fortunately, no edema was observed postoperatively. The pectineus and obturator externus muscles were severed. A Gigli saw was introduced through obturator foramen in order to osteotomize the upper ramus of the pubis.

The common iliac vessels, internal iliac vessels, and external iliac vessels were exposed. The iliolumbar vessels and lateral sacral vessels were ligated and severed. The superior gluteal artery was isolated with vessel tape. The iliacus muscle was severed on the line of the osteotomy.

The posterior dissection was then continued. The femur was osteotomized with a power saw at the subcapital line. The sciatic nerve was dissected proximally, but there was adhesion of the nerve around the sciatic notch. The nerve was carefully freed. There was no tumor tissue around the nerve. A branch of the superior gluteal artery was injured during the dissection, and was cauterized. The sciatic notch was widely exposed to the sacroiliac joint. An elevatorium was placed into the pelvic cavity, and a Gigli saw was carefully introduced.

All muscles originating from the ischium were severed. The sacrospinous ligament and sacrotuberous ligament were carefully transected near the sacrum. The soft tissues between the ischium and the rectum were carefully dissected. The tumor had not invaded the rectum. A Gigli saw was introduced around the lower ramus of the pubis. The three bones were osteotomized at the same time, and the hemipelvis became mobile. The branches of the internal iliac vessels to the pelvis were easily managed after the osteotomy was performed (Fig. 4). The remnants of the soft tissues extending between the ischium and the femur or sacrum were severed. The internal hemipelvectomy was then completed. The wound was irrigated and the sources of bleeding were cauterized.

The resected femoral head was grafted into the cut stump of the sacrum, and reaming was performed in the usual manner. The reconstruction cup and physio-hip system were implanted into the sacroiliac joint with bone cement and screws. This system is composed of a metal cup, a polyethylene inner liner, and a metal femoral component. The metal cup is secured to the sacrum or the sacroiliac joint with screws and bone cement. The femoral components are modular and are also secured to the femur with bone cement. The prosthetic femoral head and the inner liner are con-

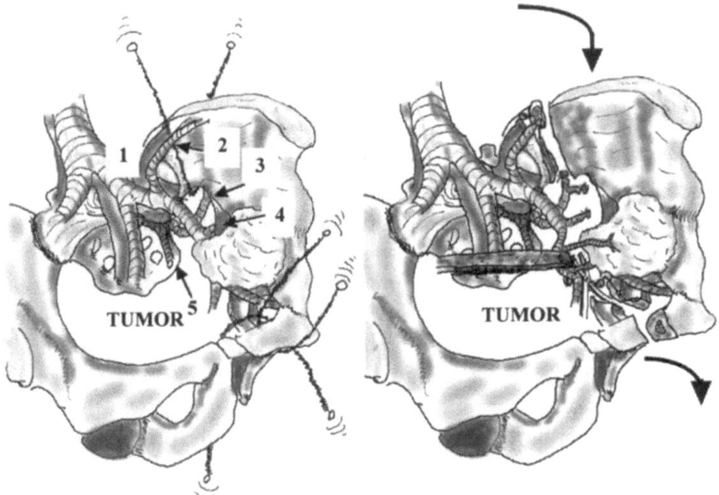

a b

FIG. 4. **a** A triple osteotomy was performed with three wire saws. *1*, internal iliac artery; *2*, iliolumbar artery; *3*, superior gluteal artery; *4*, inferior gluteal artery; *5*, lateral sacral artery. **b** The deep branches of the internal iliac artery were managed after the osteotomy had been performed

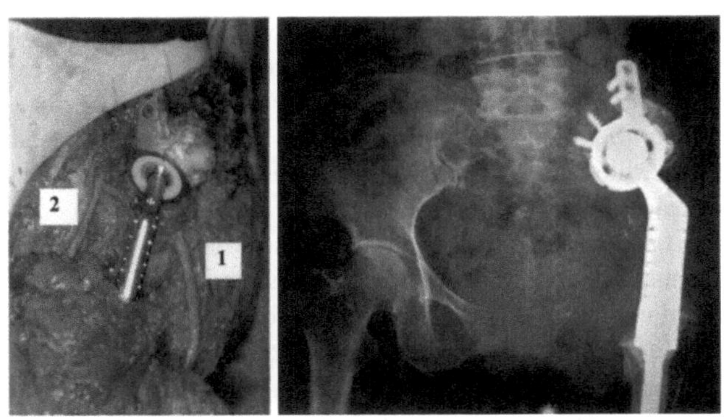

a b

FIG. 5. Constrained total hip arthroplasty. **a** The reconstruction cup and physio-hip system secured with bone cement. The cup was placed in the cut stump of the sacroiliac joint. *1*, sciatic nerve; *2*, external iliac artery. **b** Postoperative X-ray film showing the stable hip joint

nected with a self-locking system. This system is to prevent dislocation of the hip joint after extensive resection. A long-stem femoral component (120mm) was fixed with bone cement. The constrained hip joint was then reconstructed (Fig. 5). The wound was irrigated. The gluteus medius was sutured to the abdominal muscles and the fascia. The severed gluteus maximus was repaired. The wound was closed in layers leaving two suction drains in place.

The surgical stage was I B, and the margin was estimated to be curative wide.

Postoperative Course

The patient was disease-free 5 months after surgery. She requires two crutches for ambulation, but does not complain of any pain.

Case 12: Simple Wide Resection of an Osteosarcoma of the Pubis and Reinforcement of the Inguinal Soft Tissue with Marlex Mesh in a 13-Year-Old Girl

TETSUO HOTTA

Summary. A partially cystic bone tumor, diagnosed as an osteosarcoma of the upper ramus of the left pubis, was resected. This tumor was found accidentally during a follow-up examination for congenital dislocation of the ipsilateral hip joint. The defect was reinforced with marlex mesh, but no bony reconstruction was performed.

Key words. Type III tumor, Osteosarcoma, Growing child, Reconstruction, Surgical approach

Clinical History

The patient visited the pediatric orthopedic service of Niigata University Hospital for a follow-up examination for congenital dislocation of the hip joint after an absence of several years. At this time, a cystic bone tumor was detected in the right pubis by X-ray. Previous X-ray examinations had not demonstrated any abnormality in the pubis 4 years earlier. The patient had no symptoms around the hip joint or pubis.

Further X-ray examination showed a cystic bone tumor in the upper ramus of the left pubis (Fig. 1). The cortex was thinned and swollen, but appeared to be preserved. No periosteal reaction was observed. A magnetic resonance imaging assessment showed high-intensity T2-weighted images, and contrast enhancement was evident (Fig. 2).

Slightly elevated serum alkaline phosphatase was detected, but was within normal limits for the patient. There were no other abnormal findings.

The first operation was performed on April 13, 1996. After an intraoperative histological diagnosis of benign histiocytosis had been made, the lesion was curetted out. However, the histological examination of the resected specimen showed some features of malignancy. The specimen was sent out for consultation to about 20 bone pathologists in Japan, and to Dr. Unni of the Mayo Clinic in Rochester, Minnesota, USA. The most common diagnosis made was osteosarcoma, followed by histiocytosis and aneurismal bone cyst. Dr. Unni made a diagnosis of osteosarcoma. A wide resection was performed on August 19, 1996. No chemotherapy was given. The patient is currently a student, has been continuously free of disease, and is doing well without any problems 5 years after the second operation.

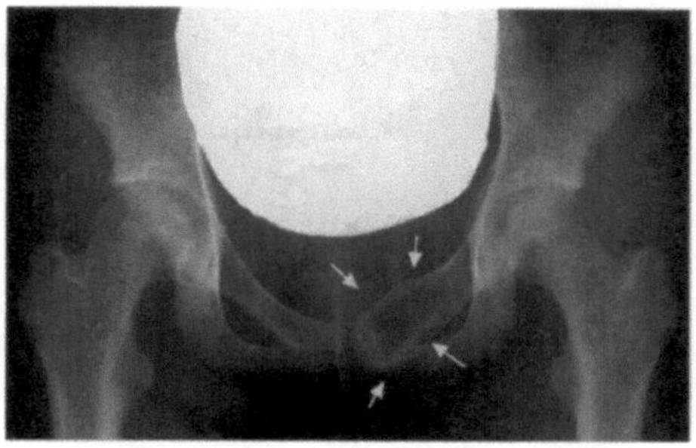

FIG. 1. Preoperative X-ray film. A cystic bone tumor was detected in the right pubis (*arrows*)

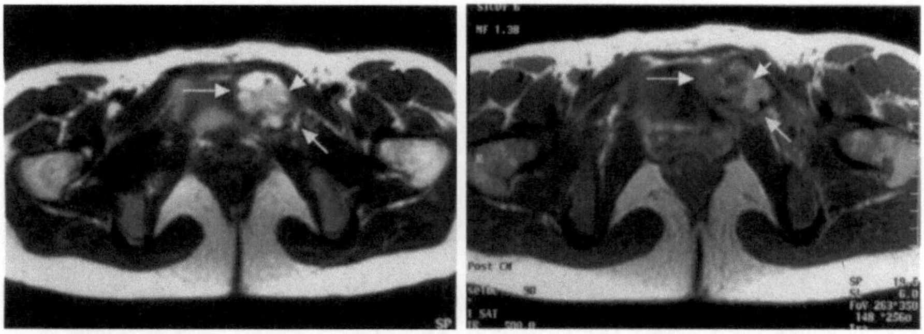

a b

FIG. 2. MR imaging. **a** The tumor revealed by a high-intensity T2-weighted image. **b** Contrast enhancement was evident in T1-weighted imaging

Surgical Procedure

After the successful induction of general anesthesia, the patient was placed in the lithotomy position on the operating table. Preoperative scrubbing and draping were performed in the usual manner. A combination of the ilioinguinal and perineal approaches was used (see Chap. 5). The previous operative scar was carefully excised in a lens fashion (Fig. 3). The retroperitoneal space was exposed first. The bladder was found to be intact, and was easily freed from the pubis. The tumor had not progressed outside the bone. The obturator nerve and artery were easily identified. The inner side of the symphysis pubis was exposed. The osteotomy line was defined on the contralateral pubic bone. The perineal approach was then deepened. The apex of the pubic arch was carefully exposed from both the inside and the outside. The lower ramus of the pubis was exposed subperiosteally. All muscles attached to the upper ramus of the pubis were transected 1 cm from their origins. The osteotomy sites on both rami of the pubis were exposed, and two Gigli wire saws were introduced. Another wire saw was placed in the pubic arch. A triple osteotomy was performed, with all three cuts being made at the same time, and the entire pubis was then resected (see Chap. 5).

The defect in the pubis was covered with a sheet of marlex mesh, as shown in Fig. 4. The mesh was sutured to the abdominal muscles, adductor muscles, and

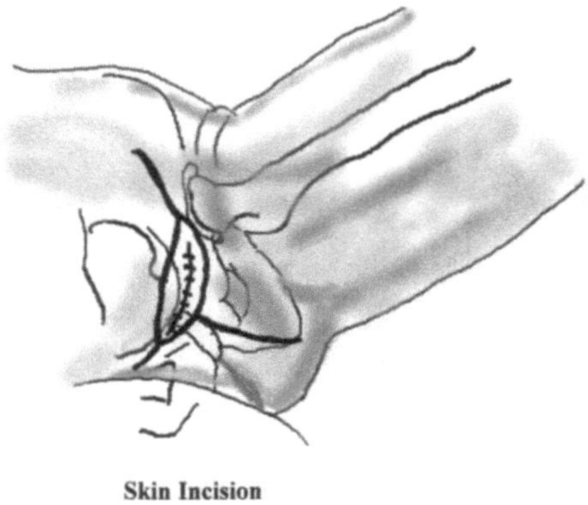

FIG. 3. Skin incision. A combination of ilioinguinal and perineal approaches was used. The previous operative scar was carefully excised in a lens fashion

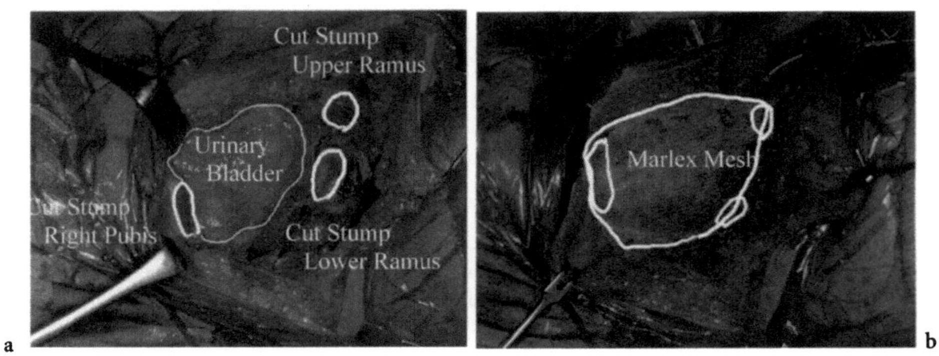

FIG. 4. Soft tissue reconstruction. **a** The urinary bladder was intact, and a wide excision was performed. **b** The defect was covered with a marlex mesh sheet

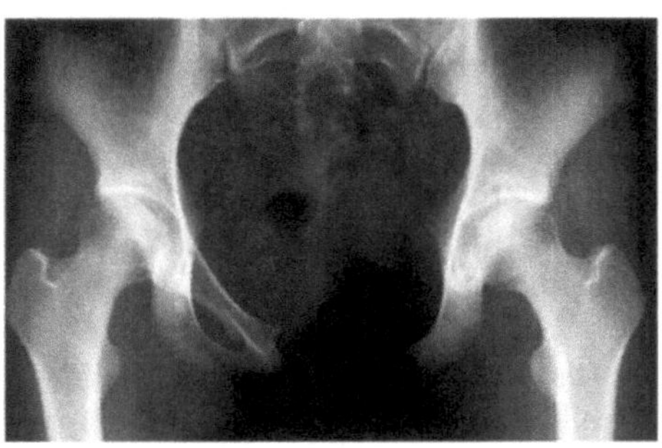

FIG. 5. Postoperative X-ray film taken 5 years after the second surgery. No deformity has occurred in the pubis

ischium. One suction drain was placed in the retroperitoneum, and another in the anterior portion of the mesh. A postoperative X-ray is shown in Fig. 5.

The surgical site was type III, the upper ramus of the left pubis. The surgical stage was II B after the first curretage, and the margin was 1 cm wide. Blood loss was 110 ml, and no blood transfusion was needed. The operative time was 2.5 h.

Discussion

The surgical approach was a point of interest in this case. A patch graft consisting of a mesh sheet was used to prevent visceral herniation. The pubis is usually reconstructed with a fibula graft in order to prevent instability of the pelvic ring. In this particular case, however, a bony reconstruction was not performed because the patient was very young, and she may become pregnant and need to deliver a baby in the future. It was felt that a normal delivery would be difficult if a reconstruction was performed and a bony union resulted.

Case 13: Crossover Bypass Graft for Reconstruction of the External Iliac Vein After Resection of a Retroperitoneal Dedifferentiated Liposarcoma in a 60-Year-Old Woman

Tetsuo Hotta

Summary. A high-grade liposarcoma of the retroperitoneum, involving the external iliac artery and vein, was resected. The artery was reconstructed with an artificial artery, and the vein was reconstructed with a crossover bypass graft using the contralateral greater saphenous vein.

Key words. Soft tissue tumor, Retroperitoneum, Vascular reconstruction, Crossover bypass graft, Artificial artery

Clinical History

The patient noticed edema in her left lower limb in February 1992. She visited a nearby hospital, and was diagnosed with a left ovarian tumor. A laparotomy was performed on March 2. However, it was found that the tumor was not situated in the ovary. An open biopsy was the only procedure performed at this time. The diagnosis was an unclassified sarcoma. The patient was referred to Niigata University Hospital, and was admitted on April 13. Computed axial tomography and MR imaging revealed a large mass in the left retroperitoneum (Fig. 1). Angiography showed the involvement of the external and internal iliac arteries. There were no abnormal findings in the laboratory data. An unclassified high-grade sarcoma was suspected from the open biopsy specimen. Permanent sections of the resected specimen revealed the features of a dedifferentiated liposarcoma. Surgery to remove the tumor was performed on April 27.

Surgical Procedure

After the successful induction of general anesthesia, the patient was placed in the lithotomy position. A double-J catheter was inserted bilaterally into the ureters by a urologist.

After routine scrubbing and draping, an intravenous catheter was inserted into the left femoral vein. Venography of the pelvis showed an obstruction of the external and common iliac veins (Fig. 2). However, collateral venous circulation was well developed in the pelvic cavity, especially in the presacral region.

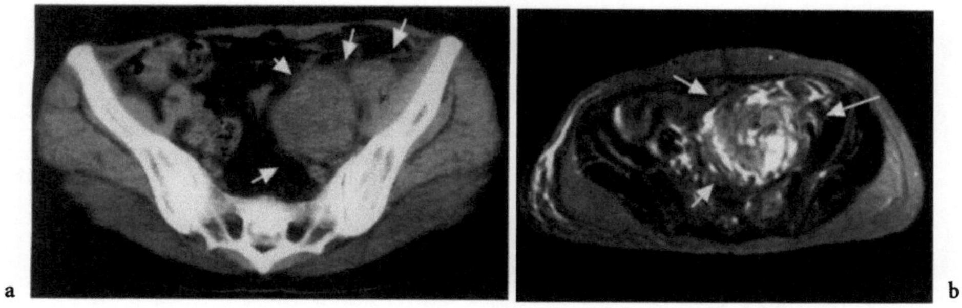

FIG. 1. A large tumor in the retroperitoneal space. **a** Computed axial tomography showing a large lobulated mass (*arrows*) in the left retroperitoneal space. **b** The tumor was exaggerated with edema, as shown by T2-weighted MR imaging

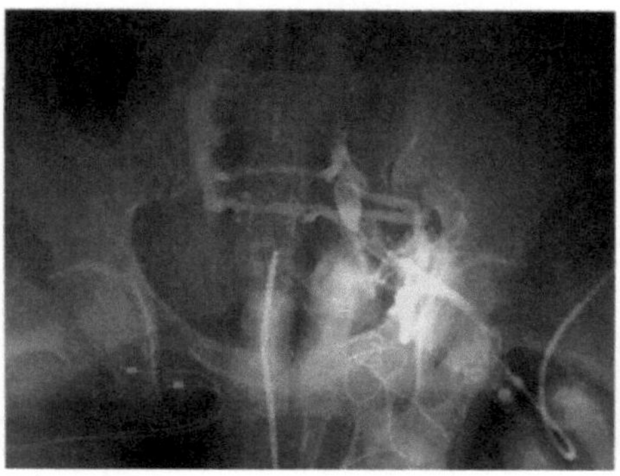

FIG. 2. Intraoperative venography showing the obstruction of left external and internal iliac veins

A longitudinal midline skin incision was made in the abdominal wall. The distal two-thirds of the incision encircled the previous open biopsy scar. A deep incision was made through the left pararectal route, and the retroperitoneal space was exposed (Fig. 3). The inferior epigastric vessels were doubly ligated and divided. A large tumor was found on the iliac vessels, which was growing into the small pelvic cavity. The parietal peritoneum was adherent to the anterior aspect of the tumor. The peritoneal space was opened with an incision in the peritoneum, along the anterior border of the tumor. The intestines were retracted medially, revealing the ovary and uterine tube. The sigmoid colon was found to adhere to the tumor. The tube and ligament of the ovary were divided, leaving the ovary and fimbriae of the tube attached to the tumor (Fig. 4). The sigmoid colon was dissected off the tumor by a general surgeon.

The external iliac artery and vein were found to pass through the tumor. It was decided to sacrifice these vessels and to make an iliofemoral crossover arterial bypass before dividing the artery (Fig. 5). This would provide a blood flow to the left lower extremity during the period of time required to resect the tumor. Vascular surgeons used an artificial vessel to make the arterial bypass between the right external iliac artery and the left femoral artery. The left common iliac artery was then doubly ligated and divided at the level of bifurcation of the external and internal iliac arteries. The femoral artery and vein were also doubly ligated and divided. The femoral

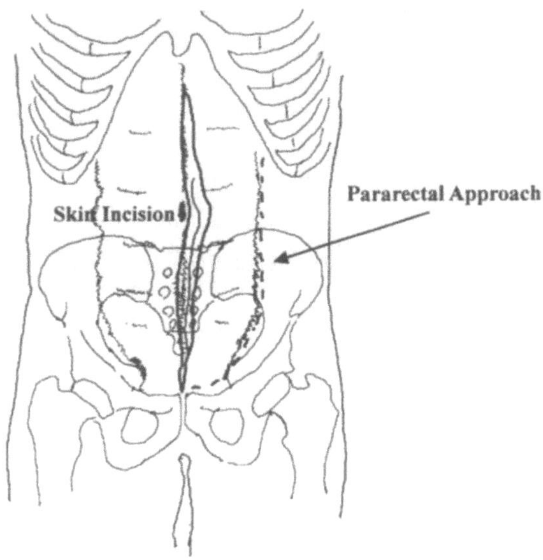

FIG. 3. Skin incision and deep incision. A midline skin incision was made, and the distal two-thirds of the incision encircled the previous open biopsy scar. A deep incision was made through the left pararectal route

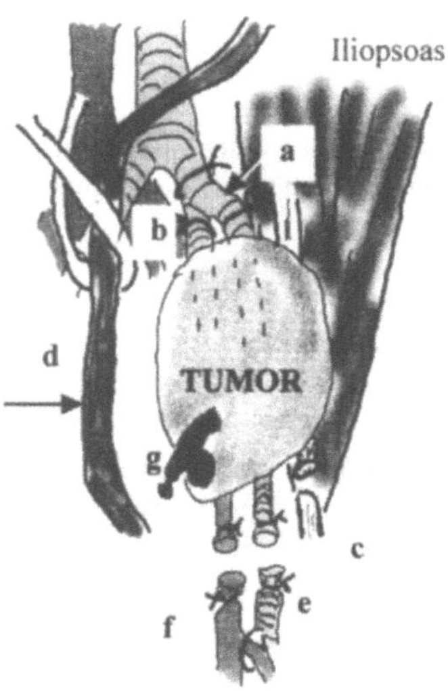

FIG. 4. Removal of the tumor. *a*, external iliac artery; *b*, internal iliac artery; *c*, femoral nerve; *d*, ureter; *e*, femoral artery; *f*, femoral vein; *g*, ovary and tube. The ureter adhered to the tumor (*arrow*)

nerve was divided at levels proximal and distal to the tumor (see Fig. 4). The thickened fascia and some fibers of the iliopsoas muscle were dissected off the tumor. The lateral portion of the tumor was then freed from the surrounding structures.

The ureter was found to be adherent to the medial side of the tumor. During dissection by a urologist, a dilated vein was found to run along the ureter. The vein seemed to be a collateral venous route, and was preserved. The ureter was also dilated, suggesting compression of its distal portion. Macroscopically, direct invasion of the

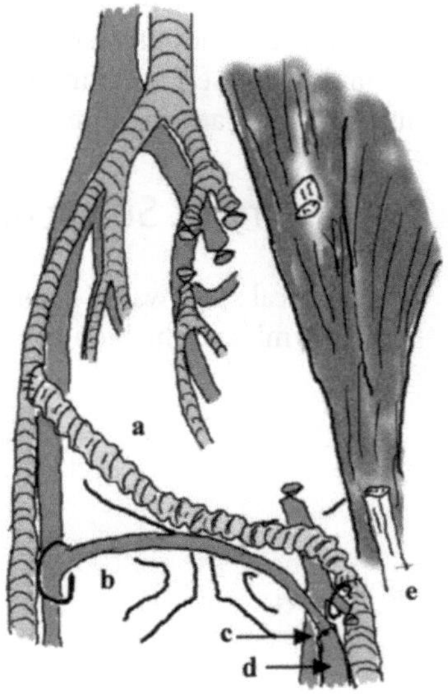

Fig. 5. Vascular reconstruction. *a*, vascular surgeons used an artificial vessel to make the arterial crossover bypass between the right external iliac artery and the left femoral artery. *b*, to reconstruct the left external iliac vein, a crossover bypass was made between the left greater saphenous vein and the right femoral vein using the right greater saphenous vein. *c*, left femoral vein. *d*, left greater saphenous vein. *e*, femoral nerve

ureter by the tumor was suspected. After the dissection of the ureter, the external and internal iliac veins were dissected. The former was ligated and divided, but the latter was lacerated, causing some bleeding. The site of the bleeding was clipped with some difficulty. During the dissection, it was found that the tumor tissue had spread beneath the aorta and the inferior vena cava. This region was suctioned using an ultrasonic aspirator (CUSA) after resection of the main tumor. Removal of the main tumor was completed by dividing the iliolumbar artery and vein, and the obturator artery and vein. Tumor tissue which invaded the walls of the aorta and ureter was aspirated using CUSA. After completing the removal of the tumor, the operative wound was irrigated with copious amounts of saline.

A venous bypass was made which drained the venous blood from the left greater saphenous vein to the right femoral vein. This was accomplished by swinging the right greater saphenous vein to the left femoral vein, and suturing together the stumps of the right greater saphenous vein and the distal stump of the left greater saphenous vein (see Fig. 5).

After sufficient hemostasis, two Penrose drains were placed in the retroperitoneal space and Douglass pouch, and the wound was closed in layers. The patient tolerated this long procedure well, and was sent to the ward in a satisfactory condition.

Postoperative Course

There was local recurrence of the tumor. Severe pyelonephritis due to obstruction of the left ureter was observed 2 months after this latest surgery. A nephrostomy was performed. The patient received postoperative chemotherapy, and a complete response was obtained for a lung metastasis. Postoperative radiation therapy up to 46 Gray was also administered. The patient left the hospital on November 8, but died from the disease 13 months after the surgery. Lung metastasis, bone metastasis to the lumbar spine, and local recurrence were observed.

Summary of Surgical Procedure

The surgical stage was II B, and the surgical margin was intralesional. The blood loss was 2800 ml, and the blood transfusion was 2400 ml. The operative time was 7 h.

Case 14: Massive Sacral Chordoma Resected by a Combination of Anterior and Posterior Approaches in a 50-Year-Old Man

Tetsuro Morita

Summary. A massive sacral tumor occupying the pelvic cavity was resected by a combination of anterior and posterior approaches. The rectum was adherent to the tumor, and was resected along with the tumor after a colostomy was performed. This experience revealed that a sacral amputation between S1 and S2 is very difficult compared with a lower sacral amputation.

Key words. Type IV tumor, Chordoma, Sacral amputation, Transperitoneal approach, Colostomy

Clinical History

This case represents a classic instance of sacral amputation due to a massive chordoma. The patient experienced an operative time of more than 18h, and sustained an enormous loss of blood (14000ml). He also suffered from renal cell carcinoma, lung cancer, and gastric cancer subsequent to his sacral amputation. All these malignancies were treated operatively. The patient is currently doing well, but a local recurrence of the chordoma and its spinal metastases are now evident 13 years after the initial surgery.

The patient experienced perianal pain and numbness in both his buttocks in August 1987. He also suffered from severe constipation in November. He visited a nearby hospital in December, and a large intrapelvic tumor was detected by anal–digital examination. The patient was subsequently referred to Niigata University Hospital, and was admitted on February 1, 1988. Imaging and clinical manifestations strongly suggested a chordoma (Fig. 1). The tumor arose from the S3 segment, and grew into the pelvic cavity (Fig. 2). It was well circumscribed, and resembled a balloon. These features are typical of a sacral chordoma. No other lesions were present in his body. We decided to perform a wide resection without a biopsy. On February 17, a sacral amputation was performed using a combination of anterior transperitoneal and posterior approaches. The patient received a permanent stoma, and lost the ability to urinate voluntarily. He could walk without any support, and did not complain of pain.

Seven years after this initial surgery, local recurrence was detected in the remnant of the left side of the sacrum and ilium. Pariative curettage and radiation therapy were performed after curettage of the lesion. Five years and 6 months later, a second recurrence was detected, as well as multiple metastases in the lumbar spine. Curettage of

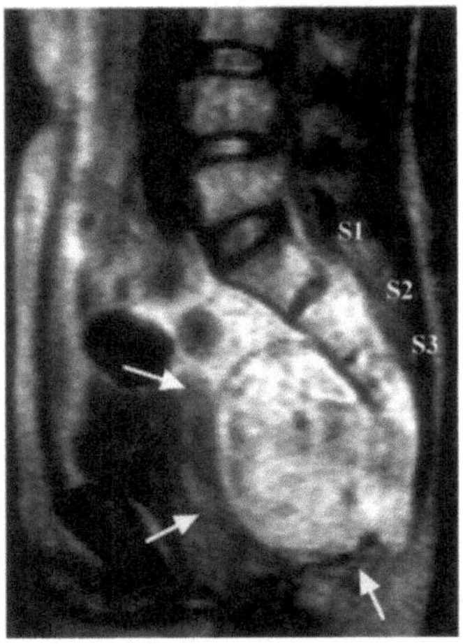

FIG. 1. T2-weighted MR imaging. The tumor showed a very high intensity image and arose from the body of S3 (*arrows*)

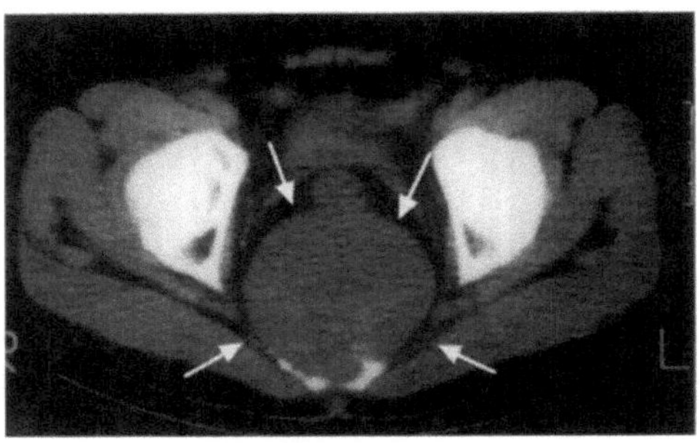

FIG. 2. Computed axial tomography showing that the tumor (*arrows*) had grown into the pelvic cavity, which it almost filled

this second recurrence was performed, and the cavity was packed with adriamycin-impregnated bone cement. The spine metastases were left untreated because the patient did not experience pain.

During these episodes, the patient had additional surgeries for renal cell carcinoma (nephrectomy), lung cancer, gastric cancer, and liver metastases from the renal cell carcinoma. He has been doing well since his last surgery in November 2000. However, he is currently suffering from low back pain, probably due to spinal metastases of the chordoma.

Surgical Procedure

The surgical stage was I B. The surgical margin was evaluated as 2 cm wide. Blood loss during surgery was 14 000 ml, and the operative time was 18 h.

No biopsy was performed because the imaging examination showed the malignant nature of the tumor, which was thought to be a chordoma. This case was actually diagnosed some time ago, and may now be a candidate for fine-needle aspiration cytology.

The sacral amputation was made using a combination of anterior transperitoneal and posterior approaches. The transperitoneal approach was used because of the need to resect the rectum with the tumor.

A general surgeon first performed the Miles' procedure. The patient was placed in the lithotomy position. A midrectal approach was made as in a routine Miles' procedure (Fig. 3). The rectum was transected and a colostomy was made. The anus was also resected as in a typical Miles' procedure.

The following procedure is described in detail in Chap. 5. The anterior aspect of the sacral promontory and the major vessels were exposed. The median sacral artery, lateral sacral artery, and iliolumbar artery were ligated and severed. Furthermore, the anterior divisions of both internal iliac arteries were carefully ligated and severed. Both S1 roots were carefully dissected and preserved, while both S2 roots were sacrificed. An osteotome was used to create an osteotomy at the lower edge of S1, which was extended as far as possible. Both sacroiliac joints and sciatic notches were carefully exposed. Lateral osteotomies were also made on both sides by the anterior

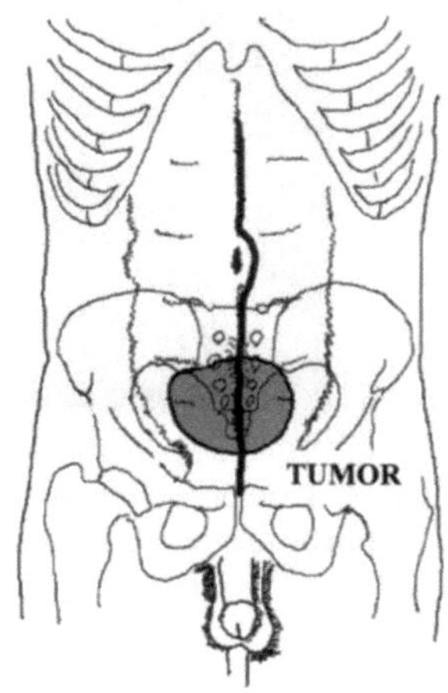

FIG. 3. Anterior skin incision. A midline skin incision was made for the Miles' procedure and dissection of the presacral area

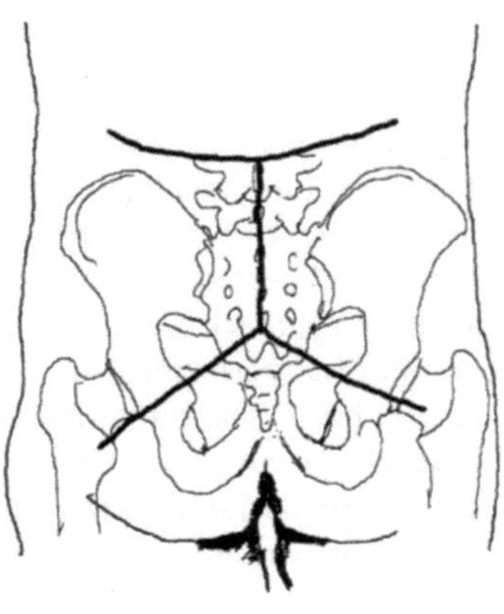

FIG. 4. Posterior skin incision. A double-door-shaped skin incision was used in this particular case to obtain a wider exposure

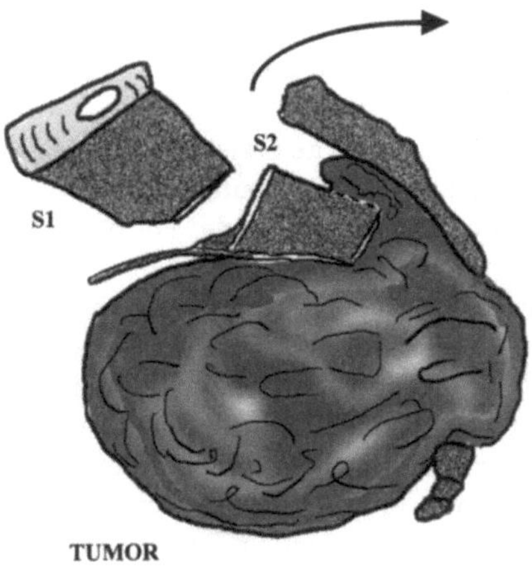

FIG. 5. Tumor resection. The tumor-bearing sacrum was retracted posteriorly and removed after the management of deep branches of the internal iliac artery and vein

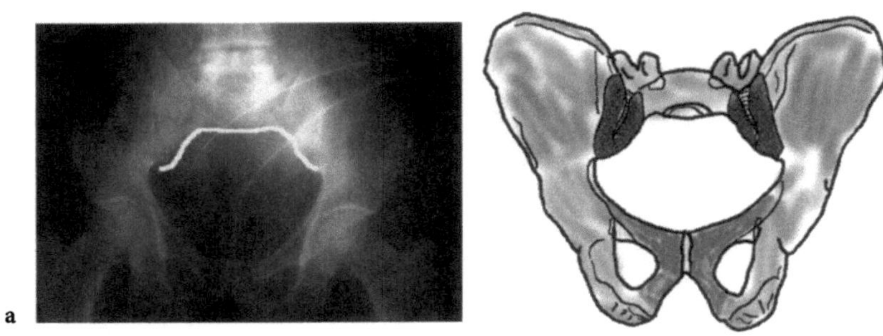

FIG. 6. Postoperative view. **a** An X-ray film showing the absence of the sacrum below S1. **b** Schematic diagram of the posterior view

approach, and were extended as far as possible. The wound was irrigated and temporarily closed.

The patient was then moved into a prone position. Scrubbing and draping were again performed in the usual manner. In this particular case, a double-door-shaped skin incision was made in order to obtain a wider exposure (Fig. 4). The posterior aspect of the sacrum was widely exposed, and a laminectomy was performed at S1. The dural tube was ligated between the S1 and S2 levels, and was severed. Both S1 roots were preserved. Both sacrospinous ligaments and sacrotuberous ligaments were carefully dissected and severed. Both sciatic notches and the osteotomy sites from the anterior approach were identified at the level of the disc between S1 and S2. A discectomy was performed, the bilateral osteotomy was completed, and the sacrum below S1 was freed. The tumor-bearing sacrum was retracted posteriorly (Fig. 5), and the branches of the internal iliac artery and vein were carefully ligated and severed. The sacral amputation between S1 and S2 was then completed (Fig. 6). Both sacroiliac joints were stable, and no reconstruction was performed.

Postoperative Course

The dead space resulting from the surgical procedure was left alone. A seroma was observed postoperatively, but was adequately treated by redrainage. There was no infection. Local recurrence and multiple spine metastases occurred 13 years after the initial surgery. The patient is currently alive, but with the diseases described above.

Case 15: Metastatic Type II Tumor in a 67-Year-Old Man Treated by Standard Total Hip Arthroplasty After Three-Dimensional Pelvic Osteotomy and Preservation of the Posterior Column of the Acetabulum

Tetsuo Hotta

Summary. A solitary type II metastasis of renal cell carcinoma was resected after a detailed three-dimensional computerized axial tomography scan was taken which clearly showed the margin of the tumor. Reconstruction of the pelvic ring was not necessary. A standard total hip arthroplasty (THA) was performed, along with bone grafting of the defect in the acetabulum. The patient had been functioning well with a cane in his daily activities, but later died of the disease.

Key words. Type II tumor, Metastasis, Renal cell carcinoma, Skin necrosis, Total hip arthroplasty

Clinical History

The patient experienced pain with motion in his right hip joint in March 1995. He visited a nearby hospital on March 27. It was suspected that a bone tumor was present in his right ilium, and he was referred to Niigata University Hospital (NUH) on April 6. A mass was palpated through the skin, and fine-needle aspiration biopsy cytology was performed without the use of an image intensifier. The biopsy revealed the features of carcinoma cells, and a renal cell carcinoma was suspected. The patient was referred to the Department of Urology, NUH, and renal cancer was detected in his left kidney. A radical nephrectomy was performed on May 24, and the patient was transferred to the Department of Orthopedic Surgery, NUH, on June 19.

An imaging examination was performed. X-ray examination showed a well-circumscribed osteolytic lesion in the roof of the acetabulum (Fig. 1a). Magnetic resonance imaging showed an extraosseous extension of the tumor (Fig. 1b). Vascular involvement was not suspected. Laboratory examination revealed slight elevations in the serum levels of carcinoembryonic antigen, lactate dehydrogenase, and alkaline phosphatase. A wide excision and reconstruction of the right hip joint was performed on June 28.

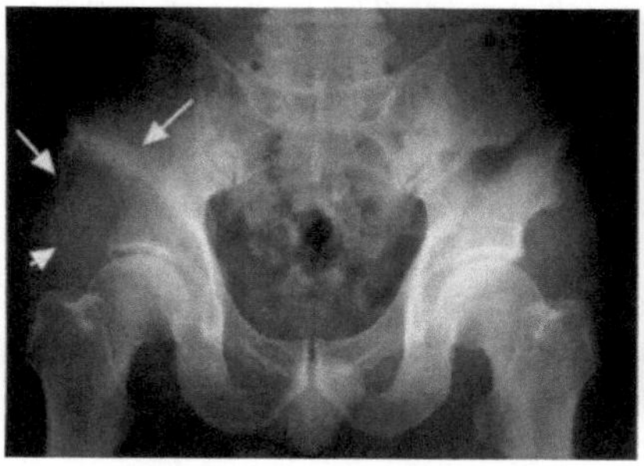

a

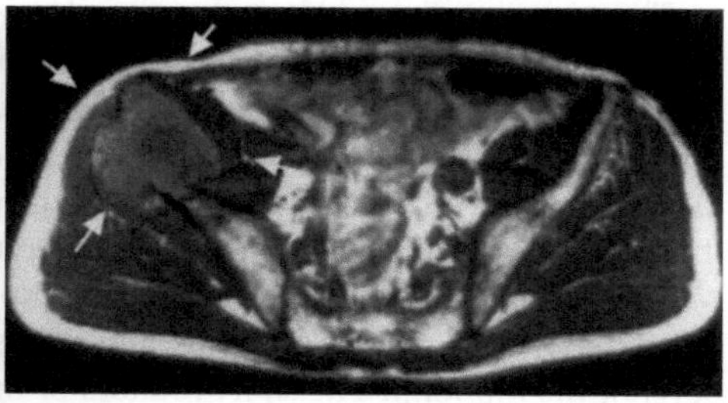

b

FIG. 1. **a** X-ray film showing a large osteolytic tumor in the right ilium (*arrows*). **b** T1-weighted MR image showing a large extraosseous invasion of the tumor

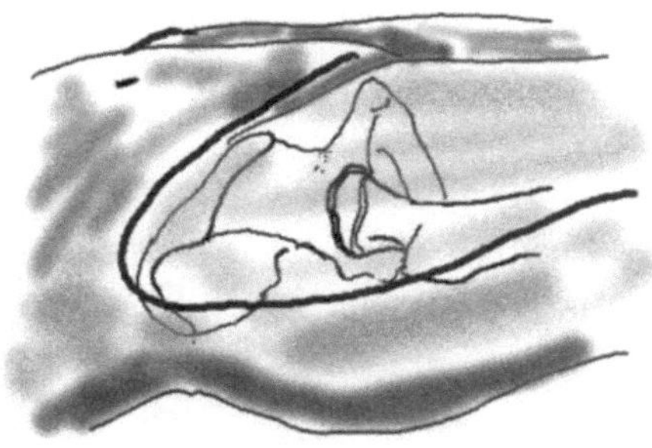

FIG. 2. Skin incision. Exposure of the lesion was wide enough, but the L-shaped skin incision resulted in skin necrosis of the edge of the flap. This experience is described in detail for the acetabulum in Chap. 5 by T. Hotta, this volume

Surgical Procedure

The surgical stage was II B for the primary tumor. The margin was estimated as 2 cm wide. Blood loss was 1800 ml, and the operative time was 5 h.

The iliacus, gluteus minimus, and a portion of the gluteus medius muscles covered the tumor. It was felt that the posterior portion of the ilium could be preserved. However, the roof of the acetabulum could not be preserved.

After the successful induction of general anesthesia, the patient was placed in the left lateral position. Scrubbing and draping were performed in the usual manner. A combination of ilioinguinal, posterior iliac, and lateral femoral approaches was made (Fig. 2).

An ilioinguinal approach was initially made, and the retroperitoneal space was widely exposed. The deep circumflex iliac artery was identified and divided after ligation. Dissection of the external and internal iliac vessels was carried out. These vessels were easily isolated, and did not adhere to the tumor. The iliolumbar artery was identified and divided after ligation. The superior gluteal artery was the main feeder of the tumor, but was left untouched at this stage. It was decided that the psoas muscle could be preserved.

The posterior iliac and lateral approaches were then made. The anterior two-thirds of the gluteus medius muscle was carefully divided from the gluteus minimus, which was attached to the tumor. The gluteus medius was detached from the iliac wing. The insertion of the gluteus maximus was detached from the femur and reflected cranially. An abnormally dilated superior gluteal artery and vein were found. They were carefully ligated and divided from the posterior approach.

The femoral nerve was identified and preserved through careful dissection. The tensor fascia lata, gluteus minimus, and rectus femoris muscles were transected at the level of the hip joint. The short rotators of the hip were severed near their insertion on the femur. The joint capsule of the right hip was excised, and the femoral head was dislocated posteriorly.

An osteotomy line on the ilium was delineated with several Kirschner wires in order to make a three-dimensional osteotomy as determined preoperatively from computerized axial tomography scans (Fig. 3). The osteotomy was then carried out with a power saw and an osteotome (Fig. 4). The wound was irrigated with copious amounts

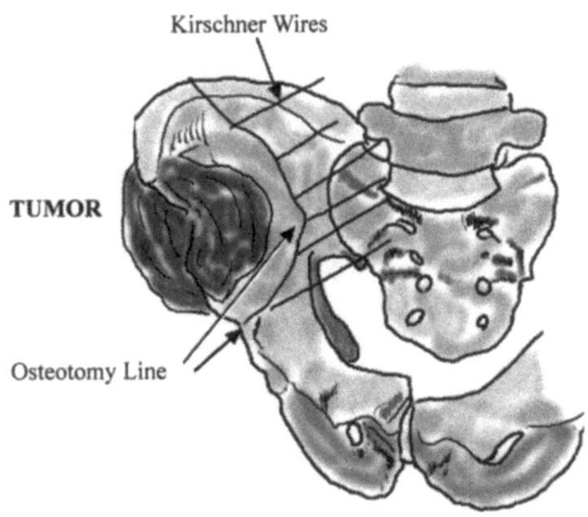

FIG. 3. The osteotomy line was delineated with several Kirschner wires in order to carry out this three-dimensional osteotomy

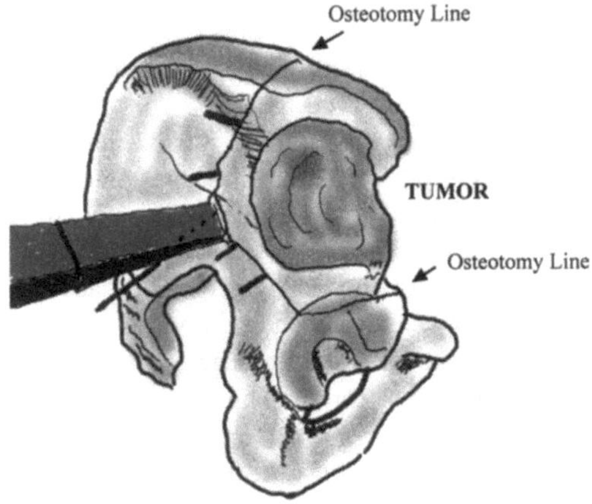

FIG. 4. The osteotomy was performed along the Kirschner wires

of saline. All bleeders were cauterized. All operative tools were then discarded, and the gowns and gloves of the surgeons were exchanged for new ones.

The femoral neck was then osteotomized as in a typical total hip arthroplasty. The joint cartilage was denuded from the resected femoral head, and a gutter was made for graft stabilization (Fig. 5). The femoral head was then grafted to the roof of the acetabulum, and was fixed with three screws. Acetabular reaming was performed in the usual manner, and a cementless OMNIFIT peripheral self-locking (PSL) cup (Nippon Stryker, Tokyo, Japan) was impacted into the acetabulum and fixed with four screws (Fig. 6). The femoral medullary canal was prepared with reamers and a rasp. A cementless OMNIFLEX femoral stem (Nippon Stryker, Tokyo, Japan) was inserted. A high-density polyethylene liner was snapped into the PSL cup. The hip joint was then reduced (Fig. 7). The gluteus medius was reattached to the ilium, and the wound was closed in layers after a suction drain was placed.

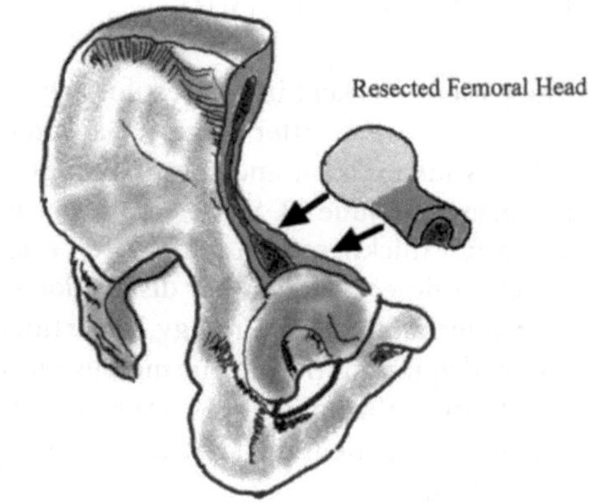

FIG. 5. Bone graft. The roof of the acetabulum was reconstructed with a resected femoral head and neck

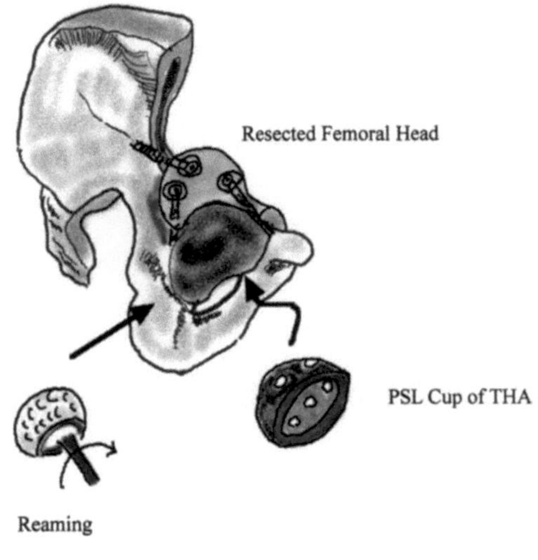

FIG. 6. Fixation of the PSL cup for THA. Acetabular reaming was performed in the usual manner, and the PSL cup was fixed on the acetabulum with screws. *PSL*, peripheral self-locking; *THA*, total hip arthroplasty

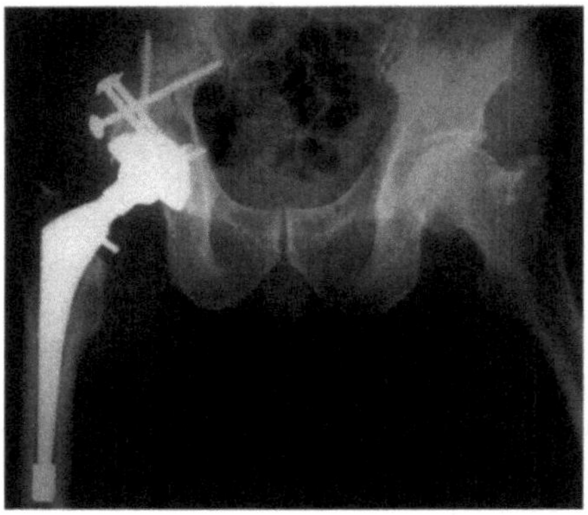

Fig. 7. Postoperative X-ray. The affected hip joint was successfully reconstructed with a standard THA

Postoperative Course

The patient was kept in bed rest for 4 weeks. Sitting and the use of a wheelchair were permitted 5 weeks after surgery. Gait exercises were initiated 6 weeks after surgery.

The wide excision and reconstruction of the right hip joint described above was performed on June 28. Skin necrosis occurred at the margin of the flap. Débridement and a full thickness skin graft were performed on July 31. The wound healed completely. Neither infection nor dislocation of the hip occurred. The patient was treated with interferon in the Urology Department. He exhibited a limp during gait due to the inadequacy of the gluteus medius muscle. However, he never experienced pain or instability of the hip joint. He walked with a cane, and was doing well 40 months after surgery. The patient then had a local recurrence of the tumor, and died of the disease 4.5 years after the surgery.

Case 16: Successful Delivery After a Hemipelvectomy in a 28-Year-Old Woman with Recurrent Osteosarcoma of the Proximal Femur

Akira Ogose

Summary. A patient with a pelvic tumor, who was treated by a hemipelvectomy, became pregnant and delivered a healthy child by Cesarean section without complications.

Key words. Hemipelvectomy, Pregnancy, Cesarean section

Clinical History

A 14-year-old girl presented in 1963 with a 1-month history of right thigh pain. Plain radiography showed an osteolytic lesion in her right femoral neck.

The patient underwent surgical curettage and bone grafting. The histological diagnosis of the tumor was a fibroma. The tumor recurred in 1964, and the patient underwent a second curettage and bone grafting. In March 1966, the tumor again recurred.

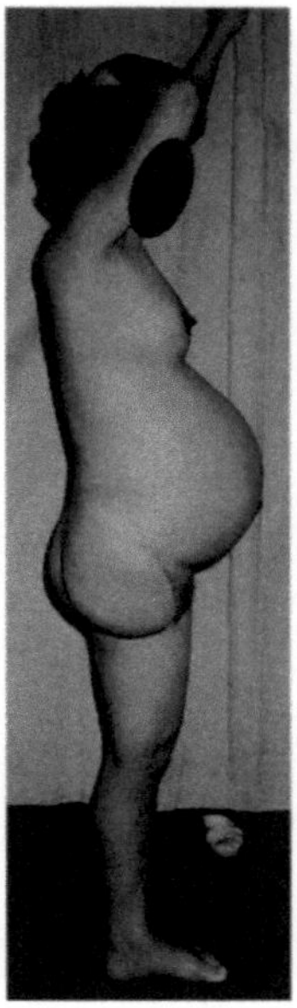

Fig. 1. A 28-year-old woman in the 38th week of pregnancy, 8 years after a hemipelvectomy

An en bloc resection was carried out, and the right femoral head was replaced with an endoprosthesis. The histological diagnosis of the tumor at this time was an osteosarcoma. In 1970, the tumor recurred in the soft tissues around the right hip joint, and a hemipelvectomy was subsequently performed.

When the patient was 28 years old (in 1978), she was married and became pregnant. Her enlarged abdomen with the fetus was supported using a special belt fixed to the left iliac crest. The patient did not experience any medical problems during her pregnancy. She delivered a healthy girl (apgar score of 10) by Cesarean section when she was in the 39th week of pregnancy (Fig. 1).

The child showed normal growth and development. The patient developed lung metastases at age 37, and later died.

Case 17: En Bloc Resection of the Entire Sacrum and L5 Vertebra for Chondrosarcoma of the Sacrum in a 57-Year-Old Man

Akira Ogose and Tetsuro Morita

Summary. En bloc resection of the sacrum and L5 vertebra resulted in long-term local control for a patient with a low-grade chondrosarcoma. Multiple complications affected the quality of life of the patient.

Key word. Total sacrectomy

Clinical History

A 57-year-old man presented with a 1-year history of buttock pain and vesicorectal disturbance. A physical examination revealed decreasing tonus of the anal sphincter, and sensory disturbance and slight motor weakness at levels S1–S5. A computed tomography scan showed a large calcified presacral tumor extending up to S1, with right sacroiliac joint involvement (Fig. 1). Sagittal magnetic resonance imaging showed a large sacral tumor invading the spinal canal at the level of L5, and extending to the S5 body (Fig. 2). An open sacral biopsy performed through a posterior approach showed a low-grade chondrosarcoma.

Surgical Approach

Anterior Approach

Six weeks after a colostomy had been performed, an anterior approach was carried out in preparation for an en bloc resection. The abdominal cavity was entered through a midline skin incision from the pubis to the epigastrium, followed by a semicircular incision at the lower end of the first incision (Fig. 3). After ligation of the iliac vessels, the tumor was exposed through an anterior transabdominal incision. The psoas muscles were severed and retracted cranially to expose the sacroiliac joint. Uncontrollable bleeding occurred during this procedure, probably from the branch of the left internal iliac vein. Gauze was packed in the retroperitoneal space, and the wound was closed. The total amount of blood loss was over 5000 ml.

The gauze was removed after 5 days, and a slight green coloration at the surgical site gave the appearance of an infection. There was no more massive bleeding. A longitudinal osteotomy of the anterior surface of the iliac bones was performed 2 cm lateral to the sacroiliac joint on the left, and 3 cm lateral to the sacroiliac joint on the

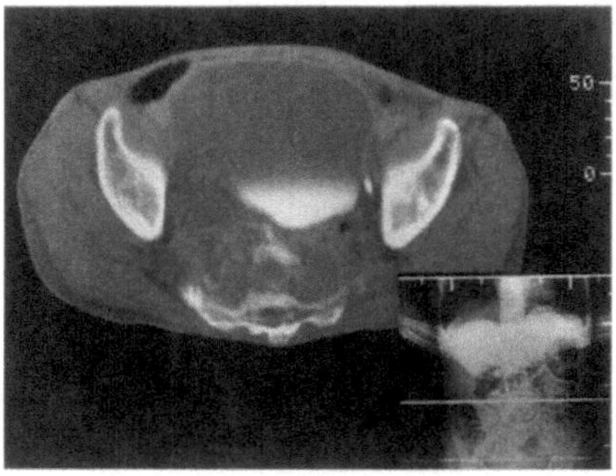

FIG. 1. Computed tomography scan showing a large calcified presacral mass predominately on the right side of the pelvis

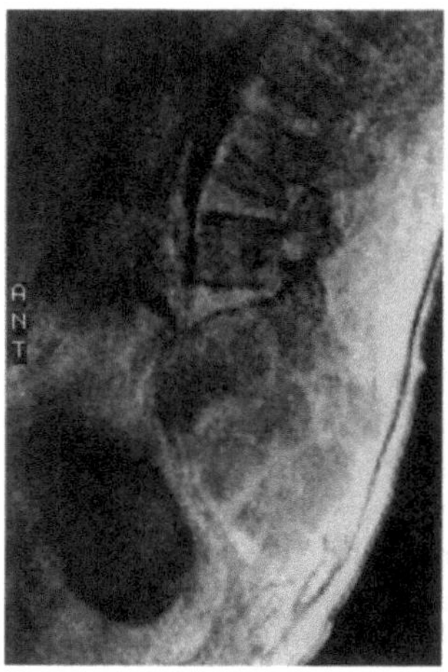

FIG. 2. Sagittal magnetic resonance image showing the sacral tumor invading the spinal canal up to the L5 vertebra

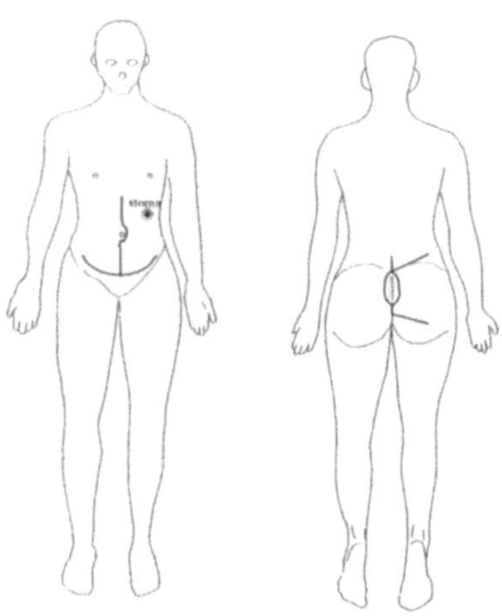

FIG. 3. Anterior and posterior skin incisions

right. The anterior longitudinal ligament and the intervertebral disc between L4 and L5 were excised. In order to prevent injury to the major vessels and urinary tract during the forthcoming posterior approach, thick gauze was placed on the bilateral osteotomy sites, the L4 and L5 spinal bodies, and the tumor mass. The wound was closed, and the patient was placed in the prone position.

Posterior Approach

A longitudinal lenticular skin incision was made around a previous operative scar, and two additional oblique incisions were made to obtain a broad exposure (Fig. 3). The gluteus maximus and piriformis muscles, the sacrotuberous and sacrospinous ligaments, and the sciatic nerves were divided. After a laminectomy of L4, a double ligation of the dural sac was performed at the level of L4–L5. The L4 nerve roots were preserved bilaterally, and the remnant of the intervertebral disc was removed. The osteotomy of the posterior surface of the iliac bones was carried out at the same levels as with the anterior approach. The sacrum became unstable as a result of these procedures. While lifting the coccyx and the lower portion of the sacrum, the levator ani was transected. Finally, the sacrum and L5 vertebra were resected en bloc (Figs. 4 and 5).

Reconstruction

It was decided to perform the definitive bone grafting at a later time because of the suspected infection observed with the anterior approach. The pelvis and lower extremities were lifted and pushed cranially approximately 3 cm. A sacral rod was inserted transversely through the ilia bilaterally, and the rods and hooks were placed between the L3 lamina and the ilia (Fig. 6). Two suction tubes were put in place, and the wound was closed. The total blood loss was 16 000 ml, and the operation lasted 13 h.

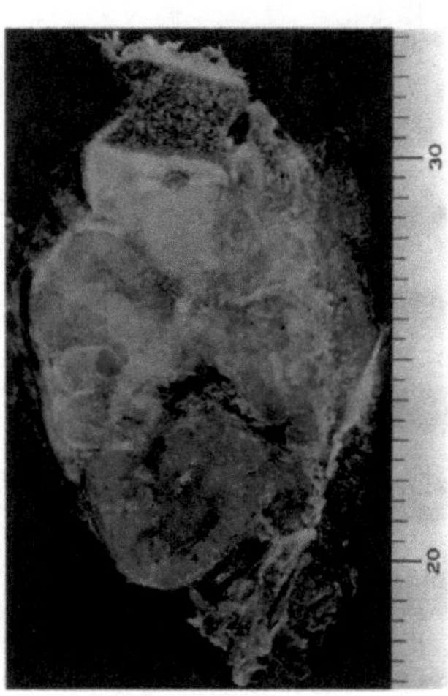

FIG. 4. Photograph of the cut surface of the tumor. Note that the tumor invaded the spinal canal at the level of L5

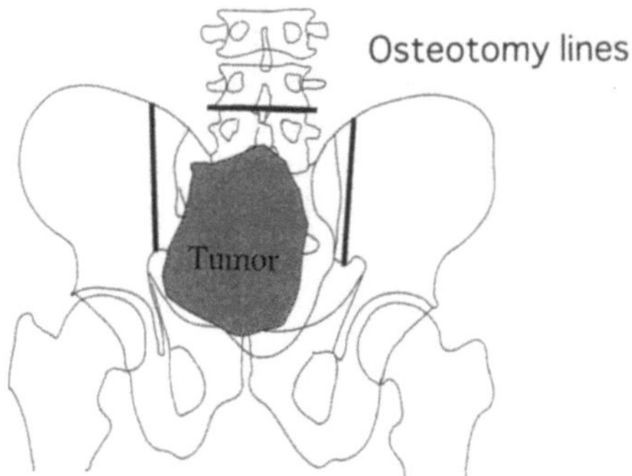

FIG. 5. Schematic diagram of the osteotomy lines

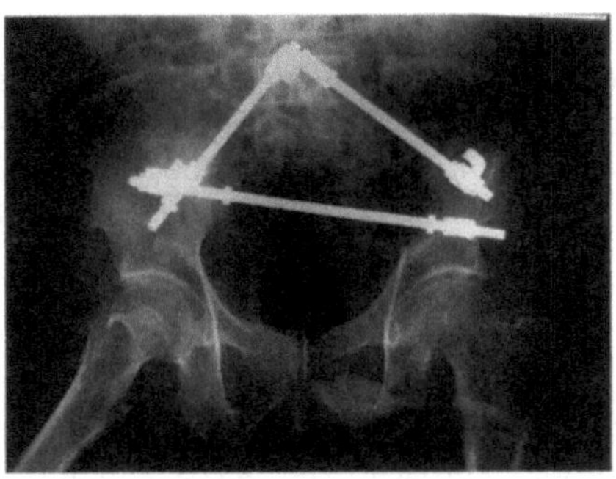

FIG. 6. Plain radiograph of the pelvis after resection of the tumor. The three rods are fixed at the iliac wings bilaterally, and at the lamina of L3

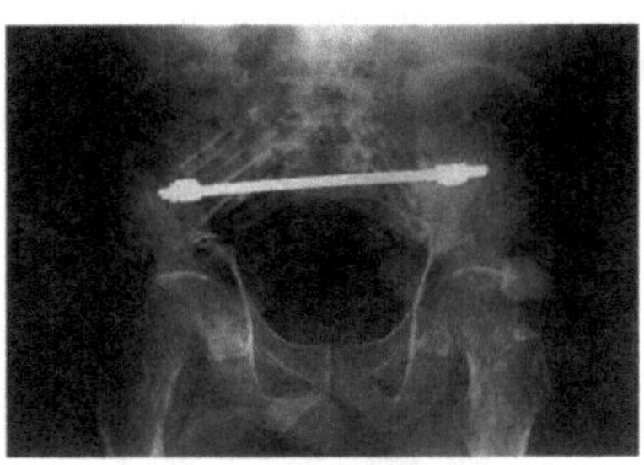

FIG. 7. Plain radiograph of the pelvis 12 months after resection of the tumor. Bony union was achieved, and the lumbar vertebrae were moved 8 cm caudally

The patient developed a deep infection (*Pseudomonas aeruginosa*), and multiple irrigations and drainage were performed. Seven months after the sacrectomy, nonvascularized fibular bone grafting was performed (Fig. 7). However, the deep infection recurred. A large skin defect in the posterior buttock was covered with a vascularized latissimus dorsi myocutaneous flap.

Postoperative Course

The patient has lived for 12 the years since the resection of the tumor with no evidence of recurrent metastasis. He can stand with two canes, although he prefers a wheelchair. He requires continuous urethral catheterization. He developed a mild form of adynamic ileus, and requires conservative therapy several times a year.

This case illustrates that complete excision of a low-grade tumor may be indicated for a massive sacral tumor. However, multiple complications may occur (Anson et al. 1994; Bethke et al. 1991; Conlon and Boland 1997; Feldenzer et al. 1989; Gokaslan et al. 1997).

References

Anson KM, Byrne PO, Robertson ID, Gullan RW, Motgomery ACV (1994) Radical excision of sacrococcygeal tumours. Br J Surg 81:460–461

Bethke KP, Neifeld JP, Lawrence W Jr (1991) Diagnosis and management of sacrococcygeal chordoma. J Surg Oncol 48:232–238

Conlon KC, Boland PJ (1997) Laparoscopically assisted radical sacrococcygectomy. A new operative approach to large sacrococcygeal chordomas. Surg Endosc 11:1118–1122

Feldenzer JA, McGauley JL, McGillicuddy JE (1989) Sacral and presacral tumors: problems in diagnosis and management. Neurosurgery 25:884–891

Gokaslan ZL, Romsdahl MM, Kroll SS, Walsh GL, Gillis TA, Wildrick DM, Leavens ME (1997) Total sacrectomy and Galveston L-rod reconstruction for malignant neoplasms. J Neurosurg 87:781–787

A List of Further References with Remarks

1. Aaron AD, Nelson MC, Layug JM, Lage JM (1995) Intraforaminal schwannoma of the sacrum. Skeletal Radiol 24:458–461

   A case report of a 53-year-old-man with a 6-month history of back pain, with left leg discomfort and paresthesia of recent onset.

2. Abernathey CD, Onofrio BM, Scheithauer B, Pairolero PC, Shives TC (1986) Surgical management of giant sacral schwannomas. J Neurosurg 65:286–295

   A review of 13 cases with erosion of the anterior aspect of the sacrum and associated intrapelvic extension.

3. Aboulafia AJ, Buch R, Mathews J, Li W, Malawer MM (1995) Reconstruction using the saddle prosthesis following excision of primary and metastatic periacetabular tumors. Clin Orthop 314:203–213

   A review of 17 cases with malignant periacetabular tumors that underwent limb-sparing surgery and reconstruction using the saddle prosthesis.

4. Acciarri N, Staffa G, Poppi M (1996) Giant sacral schwannoma: removal by an anterior, transabdominal approach. Br J Neurosurg 10:489–492

   A case report of a 19-year-old woman with a tumor revealed only by an ultrasonogram during standard gynecological examination. No neurological signs were detected.

5. Albertsen AM, Egund N, Jurik AG, Jacobsen E (1994) Posttraumatic osteolysis of the pubic bone simulating malignancy. Acta Radiol 35:40–44

   Fourteen cases of rapidly progressing radiographic, destructive changes (posttraumatic osteolysis) were reported. Primary fractures were related to mild trauma in 7 patients, and 7 had insufficiency fractures. All had concomitant insufficiency fractures of the sacrum.

6. Alvarenga J-C, Ball ABS, Fisher C, Fryatt I, Jones L, Thomas JM (1991) Limitations of surgery in the treatment of retroperitoneal sarcoma. Br J Surg 78: 912–916

   A retrospective analysis of 120 cases with retroperitoneal sarcoma. The actuarial 5-year survival rate of all cases following referral was 29%. Factors with an unfavorable prognosis were analyzed.

7. An C, Okada Y, Hamaguchi A, Konishi T, Tomoyoshi T, Kataoka A (1995) Spontaneous renal rupture caused by renal pelvic tumor: a case report (in Japanese). Hinyokika Kiyo (Acta Urol Jpn) 41:133–136

In a 57-year-old man with a history of transurethral resection of a bladder tumor 10 years before this report and vesical instillation with mitomycin C for recurrent bladder tumor thereafter, a renal pelvic tumor, a transitional cell carcinoma, was found at surgery.

8. Andreoli F, Balloni F, Bigiotti A, Lombardi P, Pernice LM, Ronchi O, Taruffi F (1986) Anorectal continence and bladder function. Effects of major sacral resection. Dis Colon Rectum 29:647–652

   The effect of sacral resection up to S2 was investigated in 2 patients with chordoma, and surgical division of the spinal roots was unilateral and bilateral, respectively. Results differed between the 2 patients.

9. Anson KM, Byrne PO, Robertson ID, Gullan RW, Montgomery ACV (1994) Radical excision of sacrococcygeal tumours. Br J Surg 81:460–461

   Four cases, 3 with chordomas and 1 with a schwannoma, were treated by major excision involving high amputation of the sacrum and lower sacral nerve root division, resulting in excellent preservation of sphincter control when one S2 nerve root was left intact.

10. Apffelstaedt JP, Driscoll DL, Spellman JE, Velez AF, Gibbs JF, Karakousis CP (1996) Complications and outcome of external hemipelvectomy in the management of pelvic tumors. Ann Surg Oncol 3:304–309

    Retrospective review was reported in 68 external hemipelvectomies: 11 cases had bone tumor; 39 cases, soft tissue sarcoma; 7 cases, melanoma; 10 cases, squamous cell carcinoma; and 1 case, giant neurofibroma.

11. Ashwood N, Hoskin PJ, Saunders MI (1994) Metastatic chordoma: pattern of spread and response to chemotherapy. Clin Oncol 6:341–342

    A case of a 62-year-old man was reported, with widespread dissemination to lung, liver, and bone following radical primary resection.

12. Baker ND, Dorfman DM (1996) Ewing's sarcoma of the sacrum. Skeletal Radiol 25:302–304

    A case of a 47-year-old man who was diagnosed as Ewing's sarcoma immunohistochemically using a marker (O 13) for the presence of glycoprotein p30/32 mic2 was reported.

13. Bascoulergue Y, Duquesnel J, Leclercq R, Mottolese C, Lapras C (1988) Percutaneous injection of methyl methacrylate in the vertebral body for the treatment of various diseases: percutaneous vertebroplasty. Radiology 169(suppl 2):372

    The goal of this clinical study was to design a new therapeutic procedure to prevent vertebral body crushing and pain in patients with a pathologic vertebral body. In 17 patients with severe osteoporosis ($n = 4$), vertebral body metastasis ($n = 6$), or vertebral angiomas ($n = 7$), the authors performed 31 percutaneous injections of methyl methacrylate. No incident was noted, and in 80% of patients a rapid regression of pain enabled a return to normal active life.

14. Bell RS, Davis AM, Wunder JS, Buconjic T, McGoveran B, Gross AE (1997) Allograft reconstruction of the acetabulum after resection of stage-IIB sarcoma. Intermediate-term results. J Bone Joint Surg 79A:1663–1674

    Seventeen consecutive patients were managed with an allograft reconstruction of the pelvis (including the acetabulum) following resection of a stage IIB bone sarcoma: chondrosarcoma in 9 patients, osteosarcoma in 6, Ewing sarcoma in 1, and leiomyosarcoma in 1.

15. Benotti PN, Bothe A Jr, Eyre RC, Cady B, McDermott WV, Steele G (1987) Management of recurrent pelvic tumors. Arch Surg 122:457–460

A review of 29 patients with regional tumor recurrence reported on the operative procedures performed, which included 3 bowel resections, 6 abdominoperitoneal resections, 8 pelvic exenterations, 8 resections of tumor recurrence, and 4 conservative procedures.

16. Bethke KP, Neifeld JP, Lawrence W Jr (1991) Diagnosis and management of sacrococcygeal chordoma. J Surg Oncol 48:232–238

Of 15 patients with chordoma, 8 that originated in the sacrococcygeal area were reviewed for diagnosis and type of treatment. Of the others, 3 were located in the clivus and 4 elsewhere along the axial skeleton.

17. Bevilacqua RG, Rogatko A, Hajdu SI, Brennan MF (1991) Prognostic factors in primary retroperitoneal soft-tissue sarcomas. Arch Surg 126:328–334

In 80 patients, an analysis was performed on treatment-independent variables (age, sex, signs and symptoms, site, size, histological findings, grade, and clinical presentation) and treatment-dependent variables (resectability, type of operation, surgical margins, surgical boundaries, microscopic margins, adjuvant radiotherapy, and adjuvant chemotherapy).

18. Blatter G, Ward EGH, Ruflin G, Jeanneret B (1994) The problem of stabilization after sacrectomy. Arch Orthop Trauma Surg 114:40–42

An instrumentation to fix the pelvis to the spine after sacrectomy was reported in 2 cases. An internal spine fixator, anchored in L3 and L4 through transpedicular Schanz screws, was attached to two DHS screws connected to each other, implanted in the pelvis.

19. Block GE (1970) Successful extended hemipelvectomy for "inoperable" chondrosarcoma of the pelvis. Surg Clin North Am 50:985–997

During the second month of her pregnancy a 34-year-old woman underwent extended hemipelvectomy for a massive, slow-growing tumor of the right pelvis, diagnosed as chondrosarcoma 5 years earlier. A solitary pulmonary metastasis was treated by a right middle lobe lobectomy 3 years later. The patient was alive and considered free of disease 7 years after the extended hemipelvectomy.

20. Bostofte E, Larsen T, Torp-Pedersen S, Ottesen M (1992) Preoperative investigations for suspected pelvic masses. Eur J Obstet Gynecol Reprod Biol 47:239–243

Of 307 patients in whom ultrasound examination was performed, 194 were operated on, 38 (19.6%) having a malignant tumor and 156 with benign conditions.

21. Bowers RF (1948) Giant cell tumor of the sacrum: a case report. Ann Surg 128:1164–1172

A 29-year-old man underwent resection of the coccyx and sacral vertebrae II–V.

22. Braunschweig IJ, Schultz S (1994) Urinary retention in infants: unusual presentation of pelvic tumors. N J Med 91:517–520

Two cases, a newborn and a 7-month-old infant, illustrated the need for prompt radiologic evaluation to detect or exclude a pelvic tumor.

23. Breteau N, Demasure M, Favre A, Leloup R, Lescrainier J, Sabattier R (1996) Fast neutron therapy for inoperable or recurrent sacrococcygeal chordomas. Bull Cancer/Radiother 83(suppl 1):142s–145s

Of 13 patients with inoperable or recurrent pelvic chordoma, 12 were suitable for evaluation and neutron therapy. At 4 years, crude survival and local control probability (Kaplan–Meier) were 61% and 54%, respectively.

24. Brun B, Kristensen JK (1979) Computed tomography in the evaluation of a pelvic tumor. J Comput Assist Tomogr 3:547–549

    A 66-year-old man was evaluated preoperatively. Conventional radiography suggested pelvic lipomatosis, but CT revealed a solid tumor without fat deposits. Biopsy revealed a poorly differentiated adenocarcinoma, probably of prostatic origin.

25. Burgers JMV, Oldenburger F, Kraker J, van Bunningen BN, van der Eijken JW, Delemarre JF, Staalman CR, Voute PA (1997) Ewing's sarcoma of the pelvis: changes over 25 years in treatment and results. Eur J Cancer 33:2360–2367

    An analysis of treatment of 35 children and young adults was reported for the impact of chemotherapy schedules, radiotherapy techniques, and surgical methods on the prognosis.

26. Campostrini F, Garusi G, Donati E (1995) A practical technique for conformal simulation in radiation therapy of pelvic tumors. Int J Radiat Oncol Biol Phys 32:355–365

    The simulation was carried out immediately following a pelvic organ opacification (POO) in 430 patients with primary pelvic malignancies who underwent external radiotherapy by means of photons at 6–10 MeV.

27. Capanna R, Toni A, Sudanese A, McDonald D, Bacci G, Campanacci M (1990) Ewing's sarcoma of the pelvis. Int Orthop 14:57–61

    A review of 42 cases of Ewing's sarcoma located in the pelvis: type I, 29; type II, 5; and type III, 8. Radiotherapy alone was used for the primary lesion in 11 cases, adjuvant chemotherapy in 20, and a neoadjuvant protocol in 22.

28. Carter SR, Eastwood DM, Grimer RJ, Sneath RS (1990) Hindquarter amputation for tumours of the musculoskeletal system. J Bone Joint Surg 72:490–493

    A review of 34 hindquarter amputations performed for malignant tumors around the hip, classifying them as palliative or curative according to the resection margins or the presence of the disseminated disease.

29. Catton C, O'Sullivan B, Bell R, Laperriere N, Cummings B, Fornasier V, Wunder J (1996) Chordoma: long-term follow-up after radical photon irradiation. Radiother Oncol 41:67–72

    A retrospective analysis of 23 adult patients with chordoma of the sacrum of 48 cases was reported, including base of skull (20) and mobile spine (5). Of these cases, 44 were referred postoperatively with overt disease, and the long-term results of treatment and the patterns of failure for the cases predominantly treated with postoperative photon irradiation were reported.

30. Cesinaro AM, Maiorana A, Annessi G, Collina G (1995) Cutaneous metastasis of chordoma. Am J Dermatopathol 17:603–605

    A 40-year-old man had undergone excision of a sacral chordoma 16 months previously. A metastasis to the skin of the nose was described. The lesion can be confused with mixed tumor of the sweat glands.

31. Chandawarkar RY (1996) Sacrococcygeal chordoma: review of 50 consecutive patients. World J Surg 20:717–719

Pain was the most common presenting symptom (82%). Aggressive resection through a combined abdominosacral approach offered the best results.

32. Choi YS, Lundy RO (1989) Rhabdomyosarcoma and hypercalcemia. Arch Intern Med 149:1189

A 56-year-old man presented with pain in his right leg and hypercalcemia (3.8 mmol/l), which was secondary to a large pelvic tumor diagnosed as rhabdomyosarcoma.

33. Chong VF, Pathmanathan R, Sambandan SS (1994) Transarticular spread of the sacroiliac joint in a chondrosarcoma. Med J Malays 49:282–284

A 35-year-old man with chondrosarcoma of the ilium presented with destruction of the sacroiliac joint and the ipsilateral sacral ala with sacral nerve involvement.

34. Cody HS, Marcove RC, Quan SH (1981) Malignant retrorectal tumors: 28 years experience at Memorial Sloan-Kettering Cancer Center. Dis Colon Rectum 24:501–506

A review of 39 patients with localized malignant retrorectal tumors—chordomas (38%), neurogenic tumors (15%), and chondrosarcomas, hemangiopericytomas, and embryonal adenocarcinomas (8% each)—was reported.

35. Crew JP, Flannery M, Manners B, Coates CJ (1995) Malignant transformation in a fatal case of giant cell tumour of the sacrum. Postgrad Med J 71:301–302

A 14-year-old girl with a giant cell tumor of the sacrum was reported to have irresectable and fatal small bowel obstruction following malignant transformation of the tumor.

36. Deramond H, Debussche C, Pruvo JP, Galibert P (1990) La vertébroplastie. Feuillets Radiol 30:262–268

The authors described techniques and indications of vertebroplasty for patients with vertebral angioma, osteoporotic vertebral fracture, and vertebral tumors including metastasis, and hematologic tumors lesions (myeloma and lymphoma).

37. deSantos LA, Goldstein HM (1977) Ultrasonography in tumors arising from the spine and bony pelvis. Am J Roentgenol 129:1061–1064

Four patients were described: giant cell tumors (2), Ewing's sarcoma (1), and sacrococcygeal teratoma (1).

38. Dominguez J, Lobato RD, Ramos A, Rivas JJ, Gomez PA, Castro S (1997) Giant intrasacral schwannomas: report of six cases. Acta Neurochir 139:954–960

Five women and one man, aged 17–68 years, with giant sacral schwannomas were surgically treated. In 4 patients surgical treatment consisted of microsurgical piecemeal tumor resection through sacral or lumbosacral laminectomy. In the other 2 patients surgery was initially performed by an abdominal transperitoneal approach followed by a sacral laminectomy with intracapsular resection.

39. Douglass HO, Razack M, Holyoke ED (1975) Hemipelvectomy. Arch Surg 110:82–85

A review of 50 cases with malignant neoplasms of the upper thigh and pelvis was reported. The most frequent complication was skin flap necrosis.

40. Dunst J, Paulussen M, Jurgens H (1993) Lung irradiation for Ewing's sarcoma with pulmonary metastases at diagnosis: results of the CESS-studies. Strahlenther Onkol 169:621–623

A retrospective analysis of 30 of 42 patients who presented with pulmonary metastases of Ewing's sarcoma treated by additional bilateral lung irradiation.

41. Duparc J, Huten D, Benfrech E (1989) Le traitement chirurgical des metastases du cotyle. The surgical treatment of the acetabular metastases. Rev Chir Orthop 75:1–10

 A study of 42 metastases, for which total hip replacements (39) were performed, reported conventional arthroplasties for minor lesions (9), and metallo-acrylic reconstructive surgery of the acetabulum (30), combined with bone grafting of more extensive lesions (8). Hip resections were possible in only 3 cases because of extensive acetabular destruction.

42. Ebe K, Nomura S, Suda H, Homma Y, Ariyoshi I, Choji T, Nishikawa E, Nakada T, Nakanishi T (1990) Intracavitary and interstitial hyperthermia with the 2-mm diameter microwave applicator (in Japanese). Nippon Igaku Hoshasen Gakkai Zasshi (Nippon Acta Radiol) 50:432–434

 Experimental and clinical studies using hyperthermia were performed on a rabbit VX-2 tumor model and 2 patients, combined with irradiation. A 70-year-old man was treated for recurrent oropharyngeal squamous cell carcinoma, which resulted in disappearance of the tumor, and a 64-year-old woman was treated for recurrent pelvic malignant fibrohistiocytoma, resulting in decrease of pain.

43. El-Salfiti JI, al-Hassan HK, Junaid TA, Khalifa MS, Christenson JT (1990) A case of isolated iliac artery aneurysm due to a malignant retroperitoneal pelvic tumor. Vasa 19:336–340

 A 45-year-old woman with an isolated internal iliac aneurysm caused by a malignant retroperitoneal pleomorphic tumor invading the artery was reported, together with its management.

44. Estrada-Aguilar J, Greenberg H, Walling A, Schroer K, Black T, Morse S, Hvizdala E (1992) Primary treatment of pelvic osteosarcoma. Report of five cases. Cancer (Phila) 69:1137–1145

 Five patients, aged 12 to 20 years, with nonresectable primary and metastatic pelvic osteosarcomas, were treated with intraarterial cisplatin and concurrent radiation therapy.

45. Evans RG, Nesbit ME, Gehan EA, Garnsey LA, Burgert O Jr, Vietti TJ, Cangir A, Tefft M, Thomas P, Askin FB, Kissane JM, Prichard DJ, Neff J, Markley JT, Makley J (1991) Multimodal therapy for the management of localized Ewing's sarcoma of pelvic and sacral bones: a report from the second intergroup study. J Clin Oncol 9:1173–1180

 A total of 59 patients with Ewing's sarcoma were entered into a mutimodal Intergroup Ewing's Sarcoma Study (IESS-II) (1978–1982) and compared with 68 patients entered into an earlier multimodal Intergroup Ewing's Sarcoma Study (IESS-I) (1973–1978).

46. Fahey M, Spanier S, Vander Griend RA (1992) Osteosarcoma of the pelvis. A clinical and pathological study of twenty-five patients. J Bone Joint Surg 74:321–330

 Of 25 patients, 2 had underlying Paget's disease, 5 had received previous radiation therapy; of 18 patients who had a resection, only 4 had a contamination-free wide margin, and a local recurrence developed in 13.

47. Feldenzer J, McGauley J, McGillicuddy J (1989) Sacral and presacral tumors: problems in diagnosis and management. Neurosurgery 25:884–891

A review of 9 cases of sacral tumors with presacral extension: 2 chordomas, 2 schwanomas (1 malignant, 1 benign), 1 each metastatic renal cell carcinoma, neurofibroma, neurofibrosarcoma, aneurysmal bone cyst, and meningioma.

48. Fukumoto T, Ku Y, Saitoh Y (1993) A new intraarterial high-dose chemotherapy for pelvic tumor using direct hemoperfusion under infrahepatic inferior vena caval isolation (in Japanese). Gan to Kagaku Ryoho-Jpn (J Cancer Chemother) 20:1679–1681

    A 75-year-old man with unresectable retroperitoneal liposarcoma was treated with high-dose intraarterial chemotherapy, using adriamycin (100 mg/body).

49. Gitsch G, Jensen DN, Hacker NF (1995) A combined abdominoperineal approach for the resection of a large giant cell tumor of the sacrum. Gynecol Oncol 57:113–116

    A 24-year-old woman with a giant cell tumor of the sacrum, almost completely filling the pelvis and extending to the umbilicus, underwent resection of the tumor in continuity with the sigmoid colon.

50. Gokaslan ZL, Romsdahl MM, Kroll SS, Walsh GL, Gillis TA, Wildrick DM, Leavens ME (1997) Total sacrectomy and galveston L-rod reconstruction for malignant neoplasms. Technical note. J Neurosurg 87:781–787

    A technique with complete en bloc resection of the sacrum and complex iliolumbar reconstruction/stabilization and fusion using the Galveston L-rod was illustrated in 2 patients harboring a large, painful, sacral giant cell tumor.

51. Gordon-Taylor G, Wiles P (1935) Interinnomino-abdominal (hindquarter) amputation. Br J Surg 22:671–695

    Five cases of interinnomino-abdominal or hindquarter amputations were reported, and 55 cases to date were reviewed.

52. Gotoh T, Miki T, Takayama H, Tsukikawa M, Tsujimura A, Sugao H, Takaha M, Takeda M, Kurata A (1995) Giant schwannoma in the pelvic cavity presenting as renal failure: a case report (in Japanese). Hinyokika Kiyo (Acta Urol Jpn) 41:621–624

    A 50-year-old man with a giant pelvic schwannoma showing bilateral hydronephroses was treated with tumor resection and hemodialysis.

53. Gradinger R, Rechl H, Hipp E (1991) Pelvic osteosarcoma. Resection, reconstruction, local control, and survival statistics. Clin Orthop 270:149–158

    Nine patients with a malignant tumor in the periacetabular region of the pelvis were treated with type IIC resection and were reconstructed using a cementless, adaptable prosthetic system.

54. Gunterberg B, Petersen I (1976) Sexual function after major resections of the sacrum with bilateral or unilateral sacrifice of sacral nerves. Fertil Steril 27:1146–1153

    The sexual function of 9 patients with severance of sacral nerves bilaterally (5 patients) or unilaterally (4 patients) performed during operations for radical extirpation of tumors of the sacrum or its vicinity was studied.

55. Hachiya J, Takenaka E, Takeda T (1973) Diagnosis of abdominal pelvic tumor with ultrasonic scanning: from the standpoint of radiology (in Japanese). Rinsho Hoshasen (Jpn J Clin Radiol) 18:601–610

Diagnostic usefulness of ultrasonic scanning was illustrated using clinical cases, such as polycystic disease, hepatoma, choledocal cyst, pancreatic carcinoma, cholelisthiasis, epidermoid cyst, cystic kidney, renal carcinoma, retroperitoneal cyst, ovarian cyst, uterine leiomyoma, bladder carcinoma, and liver cirrhosis with ascites.

56. Harrington KD (1992) The use of hemipelvic allografts or autoclaved grafts for reconstruction after wide resections of malignant tumors of the pelvis. J Bone Joint Surg 74:331–341

    A retrospective study described the regimens that offered superior functional results after a wide en bloc resection in 14 patients with a malignant tumor of the pelvic bone, adjacent to the acetabulum, that included most of the hemipelvis as well as the hip.

57. Hayami S, Adachi Y, Ishigooka M, Suzuki H, Sasagawa I, Kubota Y, Nakada T (1996) Retroperitoneal cystic lymphangioma diagnosed by computerized tomography, magnetic resonance imaging and thin needle aspiration. Int Urol Nephrol 28:21–26

    A 67-year-old woman presented with an insidious onset of right back pain. The correct diagnosis was made preoperatively.

58. Hayashi A, Maruyama Y (1992) Transiliac and retroperitoneal approach for coverage of sacrogluteal defects with inferiorly based rectus abdominis musculocutaneous flaps. Plast Reconstr Surg 90:1096–1101

    Surgical technique and a report of 2 cases. An inferiorly based rectus abdominis musculocutaneous flap was transferred to the sacrogluteal region through a transiliac approach.

59. Hays RP (1953) Resection of the sacrum for benign giant cell tumor. A case report. Ann Surg 138:115–120

    A 29-year-old man underwent resection of the coccyx and all the sacrum except one-half of the first segment after irradiation.

60. Hishikawa Y, Yoshino F, Makihata S, Nakao N, Inamoto K, Ikoda H (1978) A case of hemangiopericytoma originated from sacral bone (translated by the author) (in Japanese). Rinsho Hoshasen (Jpn J Clin Radiol) 23:507–510

    A 22-year-old woman was diagnosed by open biopsy as having hemangiopericytoma of the sacrum. She was treated with Co-60 teletherapy by 6000 rad in 6 weeks. One year later she was asymptomatic, with no evidence of recurrence except for amenorrhea.

61. Hoffman JP, Sigurdson ER, Eisenberg BL (1998) Use of saline-filled tissue expanders to protect the small bowel from radiation. Oncology 12:51–54

    The saline-filled tissue expander (TE) was described as a safe, effective substitute when no native tissue was available in 57 patients (58 TEs).

62. Huth JF, Eckhardt JJ, Pignatti G, Eilber FR (1988) Resection of malignant bone tumors of the pelvic girdle without extremity amputation. Arch Surg 123: 1121–1124

    Fifty-three patients with malignant tumors of the pelvic bone were evaluated for location of tumor, extent of resection, postoperative function, local recurrence, and survival.

63. Iachello R, Pepe F, Panella M, Pepe P, Panella P, Pepe G (1987) Pelvic tumors in patients under 18 years. Clin Exp Obstet Gynecol 14:92–96

Twenty-eight patients aged from 10 to 18 years were treated for pelvic tumor, with a frequency of 0.13% of gynecological admissions. Ovarian tumor was the most frequent type (21 cases), followed by paraovarian tumor (5 cases) and uterine tumor (2 cases); 21 pelvic tumors were neoplastic, of which 18 were benign.

64. Ikezawa Y, Shibata M, Ogisho N, Ogose A, Takahashi HE (1991) Reconstruction with latissimus dorsi flap and long vein graft for the deep infection of the pelvis (in Japanese). Arch Niigata Soc Orthop Surg 37:9

A 57-year-old man underwent reconstruction after resection of chordoma of the sacrum.

65. Isler MH, Fogaca MF, Mankin HJ (1996) Radiation induced malignant schwannoma arising in a neurofibroma. Clin Orthop 325:251–255

In an unusual case, a 46-year-old man, it was reported that radiation-induced sarcoma arose 9 years after radiation therapy for chordoma. After limited resection of a retroperitoneal mass adjacent to the spine was performed, consistent with the intraoperative diagnosis of a benign neurofibroma, foci of malignant transformation were found in areas of the specimen remote from the biopsy site.

66. Jaeckle KA, Young DF, Foley KM (1985) The natural history of lumbosacral plexopathy in cancer. Neurology 35:8–15

The authors studied 85 cancer patients with lumbosacral plexopathy and documented pelvis tumor by CT or biopsy. Seventy percent of patients had the incidious onset of pelvic or radicular leg pain, followed weeks to months later by sensory symptoms and weakness. The quintet of leg pain, weakness, edema, rectal mass, and hydronephrosis suggested plexopathy due to cancer.

67. Jaques DP, Coit DG, Hajdu SI, Brennan MF (1990) Management of primary and recurrent soft-tissue sarcoma of the retroperitoneum. Ann Surg 212(1): 51–59

A retrospective analysis of 114 patients defined biological behavior, surgical management of primary and recurrent disease, predictive factors for outcome, and impact of multimodality therapy.

68. Kaemmerlen P, Thiesse P, Jonas P, Duquesnel J, Bascoulergue Y, Lapraas C (1989) Percutaneous injection of orthopedic cement in metastatic vertebral lesions. N Engl J Med 321:121

A letter to the editor described preliminary results on 33 vertebrae (20 thoracic and 13 lumbar) in 20 patients with lytic bone lesions of the vertebral body with local pain.

69. Kaiser TE, Pritchard DJ, Unni KK (1984) Clinicopathologic study of sacrococcygeal chordoma. Cancer (Phila) 53:2574–2578

This report analyzed 63 patients who underwent surgical resection through a posterior approach.

70. Karakousis CP, Blumenson LE, Canavese G, Rao U (1992) Surgery for disseminated abdominal sarcoma. Am J Surg 163:560–564

In this report of a prospective program of 72 consecutive patients, the tumor was described as completely resectable in 64% of the patients.

71. Karakousis CP, Emrich LJ, Driscoll DL (1989) Variants of hemipelvectomy and their complications. Am J Surg 158:404–408

Of 62 procedures, 42 were posterior flap hemipelvectomies, 5 anterior flap hemipelvectomies, and 15 internal hemipelvectomies. Postoperatively, there were no wound problems in 38 procedures (61%).

72. Karakousis CP, Emrich LJ, Vesper DS (1989) Soft-tissue sarcomas of the proximal lower extremity. Arch Surg 124:1297–1300

Of 54 patients with soft tissue sarcomas of the proximal part of the lower extremity, 2 patients (4%) were treated with amputation and 52 patients (96%) were treated with limb-preserving resection.

73. Karakousis CP, Gupta BK, Zografos GC (1992) Claviculectomy for the exposure and en bloc resection of adjacent tumors. Am J Surg 164:63–67

In 11 patients, claviculectomy was used as a technical expedient for the exposure and en bloc resection of large, underlying nodal metastases from melanoma (7 patients) and soft tissue tumors (4 patients).

74. Karakousis CP, Kontzoglou K, Driscoll DL (1995) Resectability of retroperitoneal sarcomas: a matter of surgical technique? Eur J Surg Oncol 21:617–622

In a review of 88 consecutive patients, resectability of retroperitoneal sarcomas was about 95%, and the survival rate of the primary tumors approximated that of the primary soft tissue sarcomas of the extremities.

75. Karakousis CP, Kontzoglou K, Driscoll DL (1997) Intraperitoneal chemotherapy in disseminated abdominal sarcoma. Ann Surg Oncol 4:496–498

A prospective study of 28 consecutive patients concerned exploratory laparotomy, removal of all macroscopic tumor when feasible, and intraperitoneal chemotherapy with *cis*-DDP 100 mg/m^2 every 4 weeks. Removal of all macroscopic tumor was possible in 79%, but the 5-year survival rate was only 7%.

76. Karakousis CP, Perez RP (1994) Soft tissue sarcomas in adults. CA Cancer J Clin 44:200–210

The authors reviewed the cumulative experience with soft tissue sarcomas at several large centers, concerning clinical presentation, diagnosis, pathology, prognostic factors and staging, and treatment. Pelvic sarcomas may present with swelling of the leg, simulating primary iliofemoral thrombosis, or pain in the distribution of the femoral or sciatic nerve.

77. Karakousis CP, Park JJ, Fleminger R, Friedman M (1981) Chordomas: diagnosis and management. Am Surg 47:497–501

Six patients with chordomas, 5 in the sacral and 1 in the craniocervical region, were reported with review of the literature. Two patients were treated with radiation, 3 were treated with resection of the gross tumor of the sacrum and radiation, and 1 was treated with chemotherapy first, then resection and radiation, followed by chemotherapy.

78. Karakousis CP (1982) Exposure and reconstruction in the lower portions of the retroperitoneum and abdominal wall. Arch Surg 117:840–844

Exposure of malignant tumors in the lower area of the retroperitoneum, the abdominal wall of the pelvis, may be provided through the use of a lower midline incision extending at the inferior end transversely to the ipsilateral femoral vessels and vertically in the femoral triangle.

79. Karakousis CP (1984) The abdominoinguinal incision in limb salvage and resection of pelvic tumors. Cancer (Phila) 54:2543–2548

Resection of tumors in the pelvis with lateral fixation using the abdominoinguinal approach was performed in 22 patients referred from other centers following unsuccessful resection attempts.

80. Karakousis CP (1992) Abdominoinguinal incision in resection of pelvic tumors with lateral fixation. Am J Surg 164:366–371

The author described an abdominoinguinal incision that allowed in-continuity exposure of the lower abdomen, pelvis, and the groin in one field and dramatically improved the exposure.

81. Kawai A, Healey JH, Boland PJ, Lin PP, Huvos AG, Meyers PA (1998) Prognostic factors for patients with sarcomas of the pelvic bones. Cancer (Phila) 82:851–859

A review of 102 patients with localized pelvic sarcomas (chondrosarcoma, 49; osteosarcoma, 26; Ewing, 20; other, 7) was reported. Inadequate surgical margin emerged as the only independent adverse prognostic factor for local recurrence. For distant metastasis, surgical stage remained as an independent prognostic factor.

82. Kawai A, Huvos AG, Neyers PA, Healey JH (1998) Osteosarcoma of the pelvis. Oncologic results of 40 patients. Clin Orthop 348:196–207

Of 40 patients with osteosarcoma of the pelvis, 30 had surgical excision: 10 with hemipelvectomies and 20 with limb-sparing procedures. Most (58%) of the tumors were the chondroblastic subtype. Patients who had a surgical excision of the primary tumor had a significantly better survival than did those without surgery.

83. Kawano H, Toriyama S (1988) Surgical treatment of malignant bone tumors of the pelvis and proximal femur (in Japanese.) Gan to Kagakuryouhou (Jpn J Cancer Chemother) 15(4):1549–1554

The authors reviewed 93 cases of malignant bone tumor in the pelvic region. Surgical treatment gave a better prognosis in these patients, although they had a high recurrence rate, in comparison with patients with only biopsy or palliative treatment.

84. Kazantsev GB, Balli JE, Franklin ME (2000) Laparoscopic management of enterocutaneous fistula. Surg Endosc 14:87

An 80-year-old man was successfully treated with laparoscopic management of an enterocutaneous fistula that developed in the setting of prior colectomy and laparoscopic inguinal hernia repair with prosthetic mesh.

85. Keighley MRB, Grobler SP (1993) Fistula complicating restorative proctocolectomy. Br J Surg 80:1065–1067

Twenty-seven patients developed a fistula after 168 restorative proctocolectomies. Thirteen fistulae were enterocutaneous (2 with communication to the bladder); their origin was from the pouch (3 patients), the ileoanal anastomosis (3), the pouch appendage (3), and a previous loop iatrogenic small bowel injury (2).

86. Kim RY, Salter MM, Brascho DJ (1983) High-energy irradiation in the management of chondrosarcoma. South Med J 76:729–731, 735

The authors presented a retrospective analysis of 7 patients with chondrosarcoma of the bone treated by high-energy irradiation to prevent local recurrence in cases with inadequate resection. Chondrosarcoma can respond to high doses of irradiation even though the response is slow.

87. Kinoshita T, Ishii K, Higashiiwai H, Naganuma H (1997) Presacral neurilemmoma mimicking degenerated subserosal uterine leiomyoma. Radiat Med 15:415–418

A 26-year-old woman was reported to have a presacral neurilemmoma extending into the pelvic cavity. T_2-weighted MR sagittal images showed a tumor resembling subserosal leiomyoma with degeneration. CT revealed features distinguishing retroperitoneal neurilemmoma from gynecological tumors.

88. Kotoura Y, Shikata J, Yamamuro T, Kasahara K, Iwasaki R, Nakashima Y, Yamabe H (1991) Radiation therapy for giant intrasacral schwannoma. Spine 16: 239–242

A case of a 34-year-old woman was reported with schwannoma in the sacrum causing diffuse bone destruction. The tumor was treated with incomplete excision and radiotherapy and still had not regrown 5 years after the initial treatment.

89. Kurjak A, Kupesic S (1995) Transvaginal color Doppler and pelvic tumor vascularity: lessons learned and future challenges. Ultrasound Obstet Gynecol 6:145–159

In this review article on the transvaginal color Doppler assessment of pelvic tumor vascularity, the value of the technique was discussed for adnexal masses and uterine masses.

90. Levi MM, Creque LC, Cinque S (1969) Accessory lobe of liver presenting symptoms of pelvic tumor. N Y State J Med 69:1334–1336

A twisted, pedunculated accessory lobe of the liver, situated in the lower part of the abdomen and pelvic cavity, was described in a 23-year-old woman.

91. Levine AM, Chretien P (1979) Deep venous occlusion as the initial presentation of osteogenic sarcoma of the sacrum. A case report. J Bone Joint Surg 61A: 775–776

A 14-year-old girl exhibited, as the only presenting symptom, an acute occlusion of the common iliac vein. Exploration showed a tumor thrombus growing directly from a small sacral primary lesion through the local venous drainage into the iliac vein.

92. Lin WC, Lo KY, Chang HK (1991) Single-incision nephroureterectomy combined with transurethral incision of bladder cuff for renal pelvic tumor. J Formos Med Assoc 90:840–843

Thirteen cases were treated with single-incision nephroureterectomy combined with transurethral incision of the bladder cuff. There were no significant complications or local recurrence. The proposed indications were urethelial tumors in the renal pelvis and upper ureter without demonstrable metastases.

93. Localio SA, Francis KC, Rossano PG (1967) Abdominosacral resection of sacrococcygeal chordoma. Ann Surg 166:394–402

An abdominal approach through a left paramedian incision from symphysis to umblicus was used in resection of chordoma of sacrococcygeal region in 5 cases. Resection of sacrum through S2 was compatible with satisfactory anal sphincter and bladder function.

94. Lund DP, Soriano SG, Fauza D, Bower L, Jonas R, Hansen DD, Wilson J (1995) Resection of a massive sacrococcygeal teratoma using hypothermic hypoperfusion: a novel use of extracorporeal membrane oxygenation. J Pediatr Surg 30:1557–1559

The authors reported a 33-week-gestation infant girl with a massive sacrococcygeal teratoma weighed 4,000 g, but the actual weight of the infant was approximately 1,500 g. Resection was undertaken successfully, with the assistance of vena-arterial extracorporeal membrane oxygenation. The amount of intraoperative blood loss was 550 ml.

95. MacCarty CS, Waugh JM, Mayo CW, Coventry MB (1952) The surgical treatment of presacral tumors. A combined problem. Proc Staff Meet Mayo Clin 27: 73–84

The authors reported a review of surgical treatment of sacral and presacral tumors, including preoperative management, surgical techniques, and report of 10 cases, utilizing the special assets of three surgical specialties: neurological, orthopedic, and general surgery.

96. Magrina JF, Symmonds RE, Dahlin DC (1980) Pelvic "lipolymph nodes": a consideration in the differential diagnosis of pelvic masses. Am J Obstet Gynecol 136:727–731

The authors reported a review of 12 patients with pelvic "lipolymph nodes" during a period of 26 years. Most patients were perimenopausal or postmenopausal. Exploratory laparotomy was required to make a diagnosis; treatment consisted of simple removal of the involved nodes. No recurrences were observed.

97. Mannel RS, Braly PS, Buller RE (1990) Indiana pouch continent urinary reservoir in patients with previous pelvic irradiation. Obstet Gynecol 75:891–893

Use of the Indiana pouch urinary reservoir was reported in 10 women with a history of pelvic irradiation for cervical cancer, of whom 8 underwent a total pelvic exenteration for recurrent pelvic tumor and 2 had diversion for radiation-induced vesicovaginal fistula.

98. Marcove RC, Sheth DS, Brien EW, Huvos AG, Healey JH (1994) Conservative surgery for giant cell tumors of the sacrum. The role of cryosurgery as a supplement to curettage and partial excision. Cancer (Phila) 74:1253–1260

The authors recommended conservative surgery in the form of intralesional curettage or limited excision with adjunct of cryosurgery, diligent radiographic and second-look follow-up, and repeat cryosurgery in the presence of clinical or microscopic recurrence as the treatment for giant cell tumors of the sacrum. Seven cases were reported.

99. Marroquin-Nisch J, Gruneberger A, Hewel T (1995) Haematoma of the abdominal wall. A differential diagnosis of tumour in the right lower abdomen (in German). Geburtsh Frauenheilkd 55:113–114

A 80-year-old woman who was under anticoagulation suddenly developed abdominal pain, located on the right side, as well as signs of acute bleeding.

100. Masterson EL, Davis AM, Wunder JS, Bell RS (1998) Hindquarter amputation for pelvic tumors. The importance of patient selection. Clin Orthop 350:187–194

Most patients treated for pelvic sarcoma at the authors' institution underwent limb-sparing surgery. Twenty-two patients with the largest and most difficult tumors were treated with hindquarter amputation with curative intent for malignant or locally aggressive tumors of the pelvis (21 cases) or proxima (thigh, 1 case).

101. McAllister E, Wells K, Chaet M, Norman J, Cruse W (1994) Perineal reconstruction after surgical extirpation of pelvic malignancies using the transpelvic transverse rectus abdominal myocutaneous flap. Ann Surg Oncol 1:164–168

Eleven patients underwent perineal reconstruction using an inferiorly based transpelvic rectus abdominal myocutaneous (TRAM) flap for large nonhealing postsurgical perineal wounds. The primary diagnosis was recurrent carcinoma of the rectum or anus (5), recurrent squamous cell carcinoma of the vulva or cervix (4), and recurrent sacral chordoma (1).

102. Miles RM, Johnson JW Jr (1991) Giant adult malignant sacrococcygeal teratoma. Successful treatment by combined abdominosacral resection. Am Surg 57: 425–430

This report described the successful removal of the largest adult sacrococcygeal teratoma (18.75 kg), in a 58-year-old woman, that the authors could find on record. The tumor had been present at birth and had been biopsied at the time of her cesarean section 34 years earlier without further treatment.

103. Miller TR (1977) Hemipelvectomy in lower extremity tumors. Orthop Clin North Am 8:903–919

The author described hemipelvectomy based on his series of 126 personally performed hemipelvectomies, concerning indication, preparation, surgical technique, surgical problems, postoperative problems, and end results.

104. Murphey MD, Wetzel LH, Bramble JM, Levine E, Simpson KM, Lindsley HB (1991) Sacroiliitis: MR imaging findings. Radiology 180:239–244

Magnetic resonance (MR) imaging was performed in 7 asymptomatic volunteers and 17 patients with clinical and radiologic evidence of sacroiliitis. Findings of sacroiliitis were identified in 20 sacroiliac joints (12 patients).

105. Nakahara S, Itoh H, Mibu R, Ikeda S, Konomi K, Masuda S (1986) Anorectal function after high sacrectomy with bilateral resection of S2–S5 nerves. Report of a case. Dis Colon Rectum 29:271–274

A 19-year-old man underwent resection at the S1–S2 interspace with sacrifice of bilateral sacral nerves below S2 for a sacral tumor. The postoperative anorectal function was evaluated periodically for 1 year using manometry and subjective findings. Sacrifice of bilateral sacral nerves below S2 led to a feeble anal canal basal tone with the rectoanal inhibitory reflex, and a significant impairment of anorectal function was inevitable.

106. Neef JR (1994) Technique of subtotal and total sacral amputation for neoplasm. In: Doty JR, Rengachary SS (ed) Surgical disorders of the sacrum. Thieme, New York, pp 266–278

The author described the technique of sacral amputation for neoplasm, including radiologic evaluation, biopsy, adjuvant therapy, anticipated functional results, history, physical evaluation, and surgical procedures and technique.

107. Nguyen TP, Burk DL Jr (1995) Musculoskeletal case of the day. Giant cell tumor of the sacrum. Am J Roentgenol 165:201–202

Of 4 reported cases, case 1 was a 21-year-old woman with giant cell tumor of the sacrum. Both CT and MR imaging were useful in evaluating intraosseous and extraosseous extension of the tumor.

108. Ortolan EG, Sola CA, Gruenberg MF, Carballo Vazquez F (1996) Giant sacral schwannoma. A case report. Spine 21:522–526

A 27-year-old woman had large sacral schwannomas. The patient presented with a 2-month history of right sciatica and severe low back pain. The tumor was removed posteriorly.

109. Osaka S, Toriyama S (1991) Treatment and prognosis of giant cell tumor in the sacrum—study of bone tumor registry in Japan (in Japanese). Gan to Kagaku Ryoho (Jpn J Cancer Chemother) 18:91–96

The authors reported the results of questionnaire in 14 cases from the bone tumor registry. Better results were shown in patients treated by surgery alone than in those treated by combined surgery and radiotherapy.

110. Osawa S, Nishimura T, Akimoto M, Abe H, Hamasaki T, Kuroda S (2001) Repair of a fistula between the bladder and the perineal skin by femoral gracilis flap interposition. Int J Urol 8:80–82

A case was reported of a 70-year-old woman, with a history of a total hysterectomy for uterine cancer 10 years previously, who developed a fistula between the bladder and the perineal skin after Mile's operation for rectal cancer. The successful repair of the fistula using a femoral gracilis flap was reported.

111. Ozaki T, Hillman A, Winkelmann W (1997) Surgical treatment of sacrococcygeal chordoma. J Surg Oncol 64:274–279

The authors reported results of treatment for 12 patients with sacral chordoma. For local control of the tumor, an adequate surgical margin was important. Gentamycin beads may be effective to control postoperative infection of the dead space.

112. Ozaki T, Lindner N, Hillmann A, Link T, Winkelmann W (1997) Transarticular invasion of iliopelvic sarcomas into the sacrum. Radiological analysis of 47 cases. Acta Orthop Scand 68:381–383

The authors made a radiological analysis (CT or MRI) of 47 bone sarcomas that originated in the ilium and extended nearly to the SI joint: 8 of 17 chondrosarcomas and 3 of 30 other sarcomas (2 of 23 Ewing's sarcomas and 1 of 7 osteosarcomas) invaded the sacrum through the SI joint.

113. Papaioannou A, Papageorgiou G, Volk H (1985) Hemipelvectomy for neoplasms not originating in the pelvis. Oncology 42:13–17

Ten patients underwent hemipelvectomy, mainly for sarcomas originating high in the thigh, ormelanomas, and epidermoid carcinomas metastatic to the groin. Tumors treated successfully were large and with indolent locoregional growth, often despite repeated unsuccessful local treatment attempts. Conversely, patients with melanoma had a short history before the operation and died soon after.

114. Peng XW, Wen SX, Yu YS, Bo CY, Jie WJ (1990) Primary sacral tumors and their surgical treatment. Clin Med J 103:879–884

The authors reported a review of 87 patients with primary sacral tumor treated surgically. The lesions consisted of benign tumors (17 patients) such as neurofibroma, chordomas (41), giant cell tumors (21), and malignant growths (8).

115. Porter AD, Simpson AH, Davis AM, Griffin AM, Bell RS (1994) Diagnosis and management of sacral bone tumours. Can J Surg 37:473–478

The authors reported a retrospective study of 29 patients with sacral tumors to evaluate the efficacy of current treatment. Symptoms were present for a mean of 12 months to the time of presentation. Low back pain was present in 28 of 29 patients. Early diagnosis would be facilitated by rectal examination and bone scanning in patients with persistent low back pain.

116. Prabhakaran PS, Misra S, Kannan V, Chandrashekar M, Vijayakumar M, Veerendrakumar KV, Anantha N (1998) Sacral chordomas: a 10-year study. Austlas Radiol 42:42–46

A retrospective analysis of 14 patients, 13 males and 1 female, was reported. Seventy-one percent of patients presented with symptoms related to a painful sacral mass. Eight patients underwent radical surgery and two had adjuvant radiotherapy. One patient had a partial resection. Three received radical radiotherapy. Two were offered only pain relief medication. The median follow-up was 33 months, and the overall survival at 5 years was 48 %.

117. Radford DM, Walker HSJ (1992) Cross-femoral venous bypass in combination with tumor resection. J Surg Oncol 50:136–137

The cross-femoral venous bypass procedure (Palma/Dale procedure) was introduced for unilateral iliac or common femoral vein occlusion resulting in chronic deep venous insufficiency. The authors have utilized the procedure successfully in a 47-year-old man who required extensive pelvic tumor resection involving sacrifice of pelvic venous collateral channels and unilateral ligation of external, internal, and common iliac veins.

118. Raffensperger JG (1996) Resection of a massive sacrococcygeal teratoma using hypothermic perfusion with extracorporeal membrane oxygenation. J Ped Surg 31:1467

This "To the editor" correspondence focused on the temporal occlusion of the aorta before resection of a teratoma to avoid hemorrhage.

119. Rao UN, Hanan SH, Lotze MT, Karakousis CP (1998) Distant skin and soft tissue metastases from sarcomas. J Surg Oncol 69:94–98

Five cases of sarcomas from different anatomic locations that had metastasized to skin and subcutaneous soft tissue were identified in 3 women and 2 men.

120. Rogers LR, Borkowski GP, Albers JW, Levin KH, Barohn RJ, Mitsumoto H (1993) Obturator mononeuropathy caused by pelvic cancer: six cases. Neurology 43: 1489–1492

The authors reported the clinical and pelvic CT findings in the 6 patients with obturator mononeuropathy caused by cancer. In each patient, symptoms of obturator mononeuropathy were the sole presenting sign of new or recurrent pelvic cancer.

121. Rothmann SA, Schroeder-Jenkins M, Henrich L, Thomas AJ (1986) Twin pregnancy using cryopreserved sperm from a man with chondrosarcoma. Cleve Clin Q 53:95–97

A case report illustrated the usefulness of sperm banking before radical tumor removal. Sperm was collected from a 25-year-old man with chondrosarcoma. The patient underwent hemipelvectomy, resulting in complete removal of the tumor but subsequent impotence and failure of emission. With artificial insemination, the wife conceived and carried the pregnancy to term, when normal twin infants were delivered.

122. Ruka W, Emrich LJ, Driscoll DL, Karakousis CP (1988) Prognostic significance of lymph node metastasis and bone, major vessel, or nerve involvement in adults with high-grade soft tissue sarcomas. Cancer (Phila) 62:999–1006

A retrospective study was reported in 267 patients with high-grade (G2 or G3) soft tissue sarcomas (STS), which were all removed by resection (marginal or amputation). Survival of patients with primary sarcomas invading the nerve, vessel, or bone was significantly better than that of patients with lymph node metastases ($P = 0.002$).

123. Ruka W, Emrich LJ, Driscoll DL, Karakousis CP (1989) Clinical factors and treatment parameters affecting prognosis in adult high-grade soft tissue sarcomas: a retrospective review of 267 cases. Eur J Surg Oncol 15:411–423

Male sex, large tumor size, stage IIC, stage IVA, and sarcomatous skin invasion, as well as marginal excision, amputation, postoperative fever, and wound infection, were found to be associated with shorter survival time.

124. Santi MD, Mitsunaga MM, Lockett JL (1993) Total sacrectomy for a giant sacral schwannoma. A case report. Clin Orthop 294:285–289

A 48-year-old man with giant sacral schwannoma had a tumor so large that a total sacrectomy was necessary. A special method of lumbar iliac fixation was devised. Two years and 9 months after surgery, the patient was free of pain and ambulating with bilateral orthoses.

125. Scheinman LJ, Reibman SJ (1980) Peripelvic fat simulating renal pelvic tumor. J Urol 123:564–565

This was the third case report of excessive proliferation of the peripelvic fat of the kidney simulating a renal pelvic tumor. The case of a 55-year-old man, large but not obese, represented the first instance in which the kidney was successfully salvaged.

126. Schnee CL, Hurst RW, Curtis MT, Friedman ED (1994) Carcinoid tumor of the sacrum: case report. Neurosurgery 35(6):1163–1167

The authors reported a 61-year-old man with isolated carcinoid tumor of the sacrum. The histopathology suggested a hindgut cause, and the possibility of an underlying congenital tailgut cyst was discussed.

127. Schutz MJ, Fink R (1998) Localized fibrous nodular mesothelioma of the pelvis. South Med J 91:280–282

A 22-year-old man with localized fibrous nodular mesothelioma of the pelvis was reported. There was 1 previously reported case of this uncommon pelvic tumor.

128. Scully SP, Temple HT, O'Keefe RJ, Scarborough MT, Mankin HJ, Gebhardt MC (1995) Role of surgical resection in pelvic Ewing's sarcoma. J Clin Oncol 13:2336–2341

The authors retrospectively examined 39 patients with Ewing's sarcoma in a pelvic location, all of whom were treated systemically with chemotherapy. Twenty patients received radiation only as a means of local control, and 19 underwent resection with or without radiation therapy. The patients were evaluated with end points of disease-free survival and overall survival for a minimum of 24 months and a mean of 58 months.

129. Sheth DS, Yasko AW, Johnson ME, Ayala AG, Murray JA, Romsdahl MM (1996) Chondrosarcoma of the pelvis. Prognostic factors for 67 patients treated with definitive surgery. Cancer (Phila) 78:745–750

The authors retrospectively analyzed 67 patients with chondrosarcoma (CS) of the pelvis treated by definitive surgery. Thirty-two patients underwent a limb-sparing surgical resection and 35 patients underwent hemipelvectomy. The critical issue for a favorable outcome in low-grade CS of the pelvis was adequate surgical excision (i.e., negative surgical margin). The high rate of systemic failure in high-grade and dedifferentiated CS, despite adequate surgery, emphasized the need for more effective systemic surgery.

130. Shikata J, Yamamuro T, Kotoura Y, Mikawa Y, Iida H, Maetani S (1988) Total sacrectomy and reconstruction for primary tumors. Report of two cases. J Bone Joint Surg 70A:122–125

The authors reported a successful total sacrectomy and reconstruction in one patient with a giant cell tumor and in one who had a chondrosarcoma. In both patients, this treatment resulted in early ability to walk and the resumption of nearly normal daily activities.

131. Shimoda K, Hazama S, Mitsunaga H, Uchiyama T, Oka M, Suzuki T (1991) A case of recurrent pelvic tumor of sigmoid colon cancer showing partial response to lipiodolization (in Japanese). Gan to Kagaku Ryoho (Jpn J Cancer Chemother) 18:1951–1954

The authors performed lipiodolization and immunochemotherapy for a 65-year-old woman with recurrent pelvis tumor of sigmoid colon cancer using an infuser port that was implanted and connected to a catheter placed in the right internal iliac artery. Following lipiodolization, the level of CEA decreased to within the normal range. MRI showed necrotic change and regression of the tumor by more than 50%. DSA (digital subtraction angiography) revealed disappearance of tumor neovascularity.

132. Shin KH, Rougraff BT, Simon MA (1994) Oncologic outcomes of primary bone sarcomas of the pelvis. Clin Orthop 304:207–217

The outcome of 41 patients with primary pelvic bone sarcomas was followed for 2 to 13 years. There were 18 chondrosarcomas, 11 osteosarcomas, 5 high-grade malignant fibrohistiocytomas, 5 Ewing's sarcomas, and 2 others. Fifteen of the 17 patients with low-grade tumors survived (88%), whereas only 6 of the 24 patients with high-grade tumors survived (25%).

133. Simpson AH, Porter A, Davis A, Griffin A, McLeod RS, Bell RS (1995) Cephalad sacral resection with a combined extended ilioinguinal and posterior approach. J Bone Joint Surg 77A:405–411

A combined anterior and posterior approach was used for the resection of a large tumor in 12 patients (6 chordomas, 3 giant-cell tumors, 2 osteosarcomas, and 1 chondrosarcoma) of the cephalad part of the sacrum. The anterior part of the sacrum was exposed through an extended ilioinguinal approach and the posterior aspect through a midline approach.

134. Sindelar WF, Kinsella TJ, Chen PW, DeLaney TF, Tepper JE, Rosenberg SA, Glatstein E (1993) Intraoperative radiotherapy in retroperitoneal sarcomas. Final results of a prospective, randomized, clinical trial. Arch Surg 128:402–410

Thirty-five patients with surgically resected sarcomas of the retroperitoneum were enrolled in a trial comparing 20-Gy intraoperative radiotherapy in combination with postoperative low-dose (35- to 40-Gy) external-beam radiotherapy with postoperative high-dose (50- to 55-Gy) external-beam radiotherapy alone.

135. Sloan D (1988) Diagnosis of a tumor with an unusual presentation in the pelvis. Am J Obstet Gynecol 159:826–827

A 47-year-old multiparous woman with signs and symptoms of sudden, copious vaginal bleeding was revealed to have a classic-appearing aborting leiomyoma. Subsequent surgery and histologic examination revealed a rare pelvic tumor, a malignant melanoma.

136. Stepanek J, Cataldo SA, Ebersold MJ, Lindor NM, Jenkins RB, Unni K, Weinshenker BG, Ribenstein RL (1998) Familial chordoma with probable autosomal dominant inheritance. Am J Med Genet 75:335–336

The authors described a family of Scottish-Irish ancestry with 4 histologically confirmed cases of chordoma in two generations, consistent with autosomal dominant inheritance.

137. Stutley JE, Conway WF (1994) Magnetic resonance imaging of the pelvis and hips. Orthopedics (Thorofare, NJ) 17:1053–1062

Normal MR anatomy and development, MR techniques, and the MR appearances of various pathological processes were described.

138. Suzuki T, Aikawa M, Komatsu H, Tago K, Yamada Y, Ueno A (1993) A case of retroperitoneal fibrosis forming a pelvic tumor—a type of multifocal fibrosclerosis (in Japanese). Nippon Hinyokika Gakkai Zasshi (Jpn J Urol) 84:1498–1501

A 55-year-old woman showed right-side hydronephrosis caused by lower ureteral obstruction resulting from a pelvic tumor. With transdermal/transvesical and transvaginal needle biopsies she was diagnosed as having retroperitoneal fibrosis and was treated with steroid monotherapy. With an initial dose of 30 mg of prednisolone and subsequent decreasing dosage for 3 months the intrapelvic tumor completely disappeared. Because of a history of an orbital pseudotumor this was considered a case of multifocal fibrosclerosis.

139. Takahashi H, Tojo T, Morita T, Suzuki Y, Tajima T (1983) Treatment of the sacral and sacroiliac tumors. J West Pac Orthop Assoc 3rd Congr Spinal Sect 48–50

Nine cases of sacral and sacroiliac tumors were treated with excision, radiation, and/or chemotherapy. Operative treatment was performed by combined anterior and posterior approaches after Stener.

140. Temple WJ, Ketcham AS (1992) Sacral resection for control of pelvic tumors. Am J Surg 163:370–374

The authors described a surgical approach for treating patients with resected, recurrent, posterior pelvic visceral tumors involving the sacrum. Of 11 patients, 9 had rectal cancer, 1 had chordoma, and 1 had cancer of the cervix.

141. Thomson J, Doty JR (1994) Sacral biomechanics and reconstruction. In: Doty JR, Rengachary SS (eds) Surgical disorders of the sacrum. Thieme, New York, pp 253–256

This chapter described biomechanics of fractures of the sacrum and of stability after sacral resection for tumors.

142. Tomita K, Kawahara N (1996) The threadwire saw: a new device for cutting bone. J Bone Joint Surg 78A:1915–1917

The authors described a new device for cutting bone, the threadwire saw.

143. Turk PS, Peters N, Libbery NP, Wanebo HJ (1992) Diagnosis and management of giant intrasacral schwannoma. Cancer (Phila) 70:2650–2667

A 41-year-old man with giant intrasacral schwannoma was reported, and the presentation, diagnosis, and management of 21 cases in the literature were reviewed.

144. Turner ML, Mulhern CB, Dalinka MK (1981) Lesions of the sacrum. Differential diagnosis and radiological evaluation. JAMA 245:275–277

The authors described techniques to make the diagnosis with standard anterioposterior projections, bone scanning with technetium, and computed tomography on lesions of the sacrum.

145. Veth RPH, Koops HS, Nielsen HKL, Oldfoll J, Verkerke GJ, Postma A (1993) A critique of techniques for reconstruction after internal hemipelvectomy for osteosarcoma. In: Humphrey GB (ed) Ostosarcoma in adolescents and young adults. Kluwer, Boston, pp 221–229

The authors made a critical review for reconstruction after internal hemipelvetomy for osteosarcoma according to Enneking's types of resection of the pelvis and the sacrum. It was emphasized that one has to search for the simplest method of reconstruction that guarantees maximal stability. Lack of stability and complex reconstructive procedures are connected with a high risk of complications.

146. Walker RH (1993) Pelvic reconstruction/total hip arthroplasty for metastatic insufficiency. Clin Orthop 294:170–175

Four cases of pathological periacetabular insufficiency/fracture in patients with extensive neoplastic metastatic involvement of the hemipelvis were treated by pelvic reconstruction with hemipelvis pin reinforcement with total hip arthroplasty (THA).

147. Weeks DA, Malott RL, Zuppan C, Mierau GW, Bechwith JB (1991) Primitive pelvic sarcoma resembling clear cell sarcoma of kidney. Ultrastruct Pathol 15:403–408

The authors described an extrarenal neoplasm arising in the pelvic soft tissues of a 13-year-old boy that was composed predominantly of uniform mesenchymal cells with optically clear cytoplasm supported by an arborizing network of small blood vessels. The tumor was indistinguishable in appearance from clear cell sarcoma of kidney.

148. Weill A, Chiras J, Simon JM, Rose M, Sola-Martinez T, Enkaoua E (1996) Spinal metastases: indications for and results of percutaneous injection of acrylic surgical cement. Radiology 199:241–247

Thirty-seven patients underwent 52 percutaneous injections of surgical cement into a vertebra (vertebroplasty) in 40 procedures, which was a minimally invasive procedure that provided immediate and long-term pain relief and contributed to spinal stabilization.

149. Xia RY, Luo YX, Wang TP (1994) Operational techniques and combination treatment for the recurrent sacro-coccygeal tumor. J Tongji Med Univ 14:245–245

The authors reported 6 cases with recurrent sacrococcygeal tumor, analyzing the causes of recurrence, surgical technique for second-time operation, and concomitant treatment.

150. Xu WP, Song XW, Yue SY, Cai YB, Wu J (1990) Primary sacral tumors and their surgical treatment. A report of 87 cases. Chin Med J 103:879–884

The authors reported 87 patients with primary sacral tumor who were treated surgically. A total of 99 operations including 13 total and 17 subtotal excisions of the sacrum, as well as 12 for recurrent tumors, were performed.

151. Yang RS, Eckardt JJ, Eiber FR, Rosen G, Forscher CA, Dorey FJ, Kelly CM, Al-Shaikh R (1995) Surgical indications for Ewing's sarcoma of the pelvis. Cancer (Phila) 76:1388–1397

The authors reported a retrospective analysis of 19 patients with stage IIB Ewing's sarcoma of the pelvis. This study demonstrated that surgery plus chemotherapy and radiation therapy were helpful for treating patients with Ewing's sarcoma so long as the tumor was limited to a single bone.

152. Yonemoto T, Tatezaki S, Takenouchi T, Ishii T, Satoh T, Moriya H (1999) The surgical management of sacrococcygeal chordoma. Cancer (Phila) 85:878–883

This article reported the results of surgical treatment of 13 patients with sacrococcygeal chordoma. Intralesional excision was performed in 8 patients, marginal excision in 2, and wide excision in 3. Local recurrence was observed in 6 patients, with a high proportion occurring in the gluteal muscles attached to the sacrum. It was highly possible that residual chordoma infiltrating the gluteal muscles accounted mainly for the local recurrence.

Subject Index

MIX
Papier aus verantwortungsvollen Quellen
Paper from responsible sources
FSC® C105338

If you have any concerns about our products,
you can contact us on
ProductSafety@springernature.com

In case Publisher is established outside the EU,
the EU authorized representative is:
Springer Nature Customer Service Center GmbH
Europaplatz 3, 69115 Heidelberg, Germany

Printed by Libri Plureos GmbH
in Hamburg, Germany